HOW & WHY

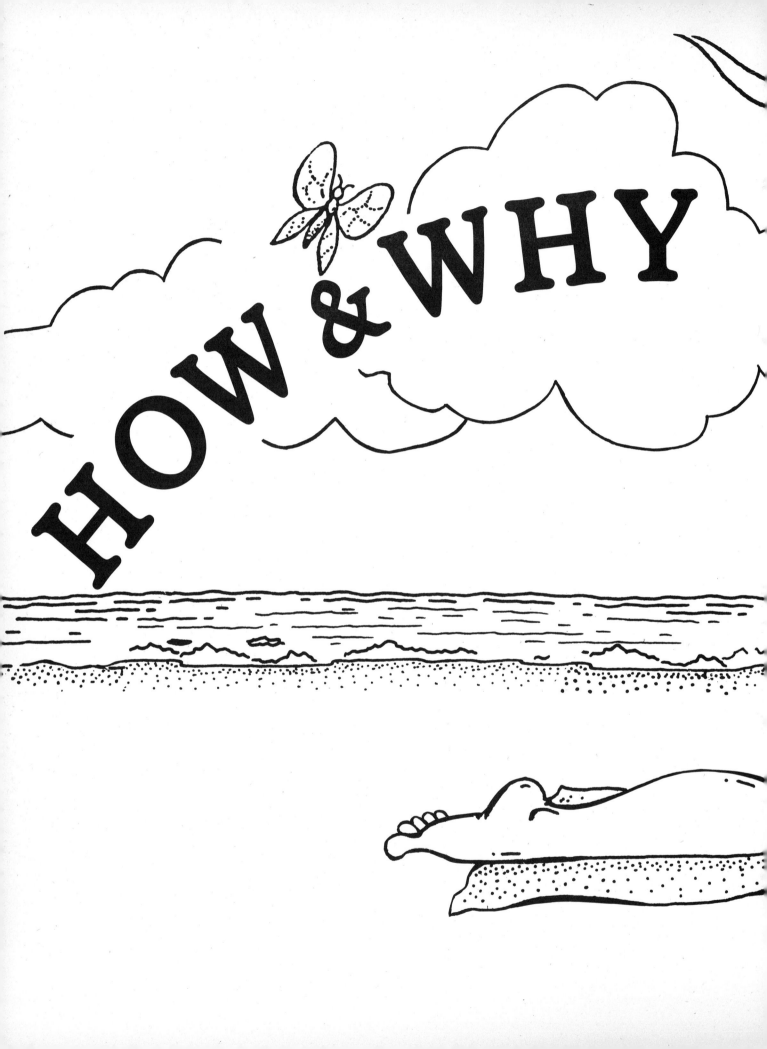

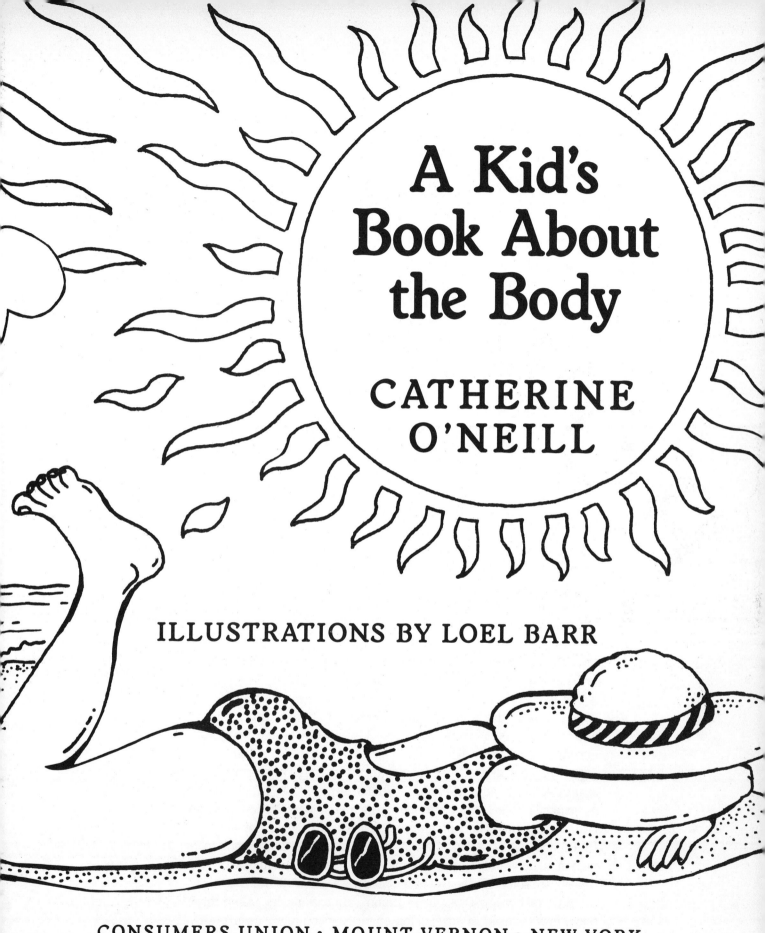

A Kid's Book About the Body

CATHERINE O'NEILL

ILLUSTRATIONS BY LOEL BARR

CONSUMERS UNION · MOUNT VERNON · NEW YORK

Library of Congress Cataloging-in-Publication Data
O'Neill, Catherine, 1950–
How & why.
Summary: Explains how the internal and external
parts of your body work, why we grow, and why we have
feelings. Answers such questions as "How does my
skeleton hold me up?" "Does my heart really look like
a Valentine?" and "Do kids get stress?"
1. Human physiology—Juvenile literature. 2. Body,
Human—Juvenile literature. [1. Human physiology.
2. Body, Human] I. Barr, Loel, ill. II. Title.
III. Title: How and why.
QP37.066   1988   612   87–71009
ISBN Hardcover: 0-89043-231-7
ISBN Paperback: 0-89043-099-3

Book design by The Sarabande Press
Second printing, September 1988
Manufactured in the United States of America

Contents

Preface

My *How & Why* project began in January 1985, when I started writing a column in *The Washington Post*'s weekly "Health" section. Many of the questions in the column—and this book—were asked by real kids who have written to me or called, or whom I have met in elementary-school classrooms. Other questions were raised by curious grown-ups. Some of the ideas were suggested by colleagues at *The Washington Post* at the paper's Monday morning editorial meetings, where such questions as "Why do I have a belly button?" have sometimes been raised alongside issues about national and international affairs.

As I have worked on the column and on this book, I have sought the help of many, many doctors—all of whom, contrary to reputation, have been glad to take the time to explain how the body works so that children (and I) could understand it. I'm especially grateful to the American Academy of Pediatrics, the Children's Hospital National Medical Center in Washington, and the Johns Hopkins Children's Center in Baltimore for putting me in touch with so many helpful physicians. I'd also like to thank my husband, Joseph Alper, a science writer. His clarity of thought and his lovely writing are a constant inspiration.

Introduction

IT STARTS with CELLS

Your body is made of *bones* and *blood* and *muscles* and *skin* and the amazing *brain* that keeps it all moving. But have you ever wondered what bone and blood and muscle and skin and the brain are made of?

Everything in your body is made of *cells.* The cell is the basic unit of life for all living things. Trillions of different kinds of cells form your body. Muscle cells, nerve cells, blood cells, skin cells, bone cells, and brain cells work together to keep you alive.

Cells get the raw materials they need for energy from the food you eat and the air you breathe. Although your cells come in different shapes and sizes, they all have certain things in common. Each cell has a thin coating, or *membrane,* to hold it together. Inside, the cell has many complex structures designed to burn energy, spur growth, or do the other jobs that cells specialize in.

Most cells are so small that you can't see them without a microscope. You grew from a single cell inside your mother's body. Called an *ovum,* or egg cell, it wasn't even as big as the period at the end of this sentence. A *sperm* cell from your father joined up with the ovum. Then that fertilized cell divided, and divided again, and you began to look like a human being. Your cells keep reproducing as you grow up.

Cells have many different jobs to do in the body. Muscle cells contract, or squeeze together, to produce movement. Red blood cells carry oxygen through your blood. Nerve cells send messages back and forth between your body and your brain.

As you read this book, you will run into the word *cell* many times. That's because anything your body does—from repairing a broken arm to digesting a Thanksgiving meal—involves the cells.

Using your brain, for example, involves cells. Some of the brain's cells are called *neurons*. They transmit messages. Other brain cells, called *glia cells,* support and protect the neurons and provide them with nourishment. You have about 100 billion glia cells in your brain!

Your brain is the most complicated organ you have. It has many different parts, which scientists are only beginning to understand. Your brain is the control center for movement. It allows you to use your five senses—*sight, hearing, feeling, smelling,* and *tasting.* It does your dreaming for you, and remembers an amazing variety of things, including things such as your best friend's phone number, the particular fresh, salty smell of your grandmother's beach house, and your history assignment for next Friday. It does your math homework, and makes up stories for your creative writing class. It invents games, laughs at jokes, and makes you cry at sad movies. It feels love.

And your brain prompts you to ask questions—such as *"How?"* and *"Why?"* That's what this book is all about. It will help you find out how your body is put together, and what goes on inside it. You'll discover how your senses work, why you sometimes get sick, and how you get well. And you'll learn why your body and feelings change as you grow up.

1

SKIN and BONES

Each human body comes with some basic equipment. Bones and muscles form the physical structure. Skin covers the body and holds it together. This chapter answers some questions about how these parts of the body are put together, and why they work the way they do.

How does my skeleton hold me up?

If you have ever watched a building going up, you know that the structure has a framework of wood or metal to support it. The skeleton is the framework of the body. It provides a structure for the muscles to attach to. The skeleton is more than a framework, however. Like the walls of a house, the skeleton protects your internal organs such as your heart and lungs. And your skeleton is designed to keep you moving.

You're constantly on the move. Here are just a few of the things your body might do in a day: scrub your back in the shower, lift a glass of orange juice, walk to school, open doors, write a list of

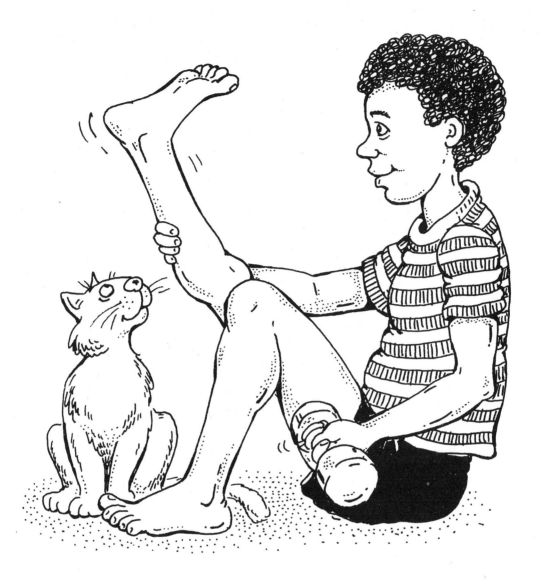

spelling words, fly a kite, ride a bike, play a piano, stir a stew, wind a clock, climb the stairs, turn the pages of a book, and pull up the covers as you crawl into bed. The list could go on and on.

You probably don't think about most of the ways you move, because you do them automatically. Luckily, once you have learned a skill, you don't have to think much about how to walk or hold a pencil or button a shirt. If you had to worry about such things, you wouldn't have time for anything else.

The bony skeleton hidden under your skin helps you make all those movements.

The skeleton of a mature human body has about two hundred separate bones in it. Many of the bones are very small. They have to be—that's what makes it possible to make small motions such as typing a letter or scratching your ear.

The *spine,* or backbone, is the center of the skeleton. There are more than twenty bones stacked one on top of the other in the spine. They fit together to make the column that forms your *neck* and *back.* Your *skull* sits on top of your backbone, fitted on like a ring on a peg so that you can nod your head, turn it, or look up and down.

Your *ribs* also attach to your spine. So do the *shoulder blades* and *collarbone,* which in turn connect to your *arms.* Your spine connects to your *pelvic girdle*—bones that form the hips—and it connects with your *legs.* You fit together like a well-designed puzzle.

You probably think of your bones as dry, brittle things. They're not. Blood circulates through a network of vessels in the bone, providing nutrients to form new tissue. To be healthy, bones must be moist. And like the rest of you, they need exercise to stay strong. Doctors know that people who stay in bed for a long time experience bone loss—their inactive skeletons actually start to waste away. Weightlessness seems to have the same effect; after astronauts returned from a long space mission aboard *Skylab,* doctors found that their heel bones had become less dense.

If all the bones in the skeleton were cemented together, you'd move pretty stiffly—if you could move at all. But the skeleton allows movement for everything from turning over in bed to doing a swan dive, because it has *joints* where the bones link up. Your body comes equipped with different kinds of joints for different uses. Some are hinges, such as the *knees* and *elbows.* They allow movement in one direction for chores such as lifting. In the shoulders and hips, you have *ball-and-socket joints.* These allow you to rotate your arms and legs around in nearly all directions. *Saddle joints* in the ankles let you lean forward or backward or stand on your toes.

Where bones link up at a joint, flexible bands of tissue called *ligaments* hold them together. Ligaments are sort of like rubber bands—they stretch to allow some movement, but they also hold things together. Another kind of tissue, called *cartilage,* is also found at the joints. (If you're wondering what cartilage feels like, feel the tip of your nose. It's made of cartilage.) Cartilage provides padding where the bones meet. It's tough, but it's smooth.

If you were building a movable human body and started with the skeleton, you'd finish Phase One of your construction project when you got all those bones linked up with cartilage and ligaments. In Phase Two, you'd add the muscles.

I hit my elbow and it felt weird. How come people call it the "funny bone"?

When you bang your elbow, you also bang a nerve underneath it. This nerve—called the *ulnar nerve*—sends a distress signal shooting to your brain. That's what causes that tingling sensation. It's not very funny to feel it. People probably call the elbow the "funny bone" for a different reason. The name of the long bone in your upper arm is the *humerus.* When you bang your elbow, you're banging the lower end of the humerus bone. Maybe that's what gave the elbow the nickname "humorous," or "funny" bone. Even so, it's not very humorous to bang your humerus.

6

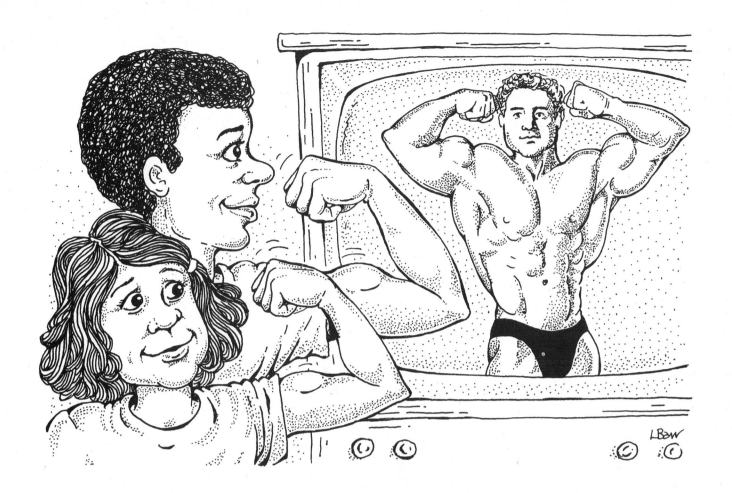

I shoveled snow out of the driveway, and now my muscles ache. How come?

If you get a lot of exercise suddenly—by shoveling out a driveway after a big snowstorm, for example—you may feel parts of your body that you take for granted most of the time: your muscles. All that bending and lifting and plowing through knee-high drifts can leave your muscles tired and sore.

Muscles need exercise—but within limits. A good exercise program for the muscles should begin with stretching and warm-up. This prepares the muscles for hard work, and gradually increases the blood supply they need to produce energy.

When you do a tough job in short bursts—such as shoveling the driveway—you may forget to warm up and stretch first. The result

7

may be stiff, sore muscles afterward. If that happens, a warm bath, a massage, and taking a couple of days off from strenuous exercise will help your muscles recover.

You have three kinds of muscle in your body: *cardiac muscle, smooth muscle,* and *skeletal muscle.*

Your cardiac muscle forms your heart and does the vital job of pumping blood through your veins.

Smooth muscle does involuntary movement—the things your body does over which you have no control. Smooth muscle moves your food through your stomach and intestines, for instance.

Skeletal muscle moves your skeleton. This kind of muscle is voluntary, or under your control. Your brain communicates with these muscles through your nerves. The brain can send many, many nerve signals at once to move the hundreds of voluntary muscles you use every day.

Skeletal muscle is sometimes called *striped muscle* for the red-and-white coloring of the fibers that form it. This kind of muscle performs activities such as walking, climbing stairs, and doing push-ups. Skeletal muscle in your legs, neck, and back holds you upright. Soon after you are born you learn to control these muscles, gradually figuring out how to lift up your head, hold a spoon and a cup, and walk. Later on, you learn more delicate skills such as tying your shoes or playing the piano.

Your muscles provide the energy that moves the skeleton. Some muscles attach directly to bones. Other muscles are connected to the skeleton by tough bands called *tendons.* Your muscles act on your bones sort of like strings moving a puppet. When a puppeteer moves the strings attached to a puppet's legs, it dances. When your leg muscles contract, they shorten, pull on your bones, and you dance—or walk or run.

Muscles work in pairs. Each joint in your body is operated by two muscles. When you raise a snow shovel, for example, a muscle in your arm called the *biceps* contracts, and your arm lifts or flexes. To lower the arm, the *triceps*—the biceps' partner—contracts. You can feel the biceps and triceps muscles bulge if you place one hand on your upper arm and then raise and lower the bottom half of your arm. That's called flexing your muscles.

There are some other places on the body where you can feel the muscles working. Try clenching your jaw by squeezing your teeth together. At the same time, feel your temples—the sides of your head up above your ears. You'll feel the jaw muscles bulge. Wiggle your foot, and the calf muscle on the back of your leg below your knee will flex. You'll find other ones, too.

If you helped shovel your driveway last winter, you probably got pretty hot from the effort. Even if you were shivering when you started, you were probably sweating inside your heavy coat by the time the job was done. Muscles use up energy when they move. They release heat in the process. That's why exercise warms you up.

If you really shoveled hard, you may have been panting for breath after a while. As you panted, you breathed in extra oxygen from the air. Your muscles needed the oxygen to keep going. The energy for muscle movement comes from a combination of *glucose,* a kind of sugar stored in your muscle, and the *oxygen* in your blood. When you work really hard, your need for energy gets ahead of your supply of oxygen. You breathe deeper to build the supply back up.

Exercise such as shoveling or playing volleyball builds up your muscles. Each muscle is made out of bundles of fiber. When you get a lot of exercise, the fibers grow, and the muscle gets bulkier. When you stop exercising, the muscles shrink again.

How does my brain tell my legs to move when I go for a walk?

Walking is one of those things you don't have to think about—it just happens. You don't have to decide to put one foot in front of the other to move forward, or think how to bend your knees. Your body does the job for you.

To walk, your brain and nerves cooperate with your muscles and bones to carry you forward. Doctors call this team the *neuromusculoskeletal system.*

Your skeleton is your body's support system, like the beams and girders that shape a building. Without it, you'd be a bag of skin and tissue, rather like a jellyfish. Your muscles attach to your bones. Muscles contract, or squeeze, to pull on your bones and cause movement.

But how do you know when to squeeze your muscles? When your mom says, "Why don't you go for a walk?" you don't have to think, "Okay, now I put one foot forward, bend the knee, swing my arm a bit, and then do the same thing on the other side." If you had to do that, you'd find it hard to get from one side of a room to the other.

The act of walking involves more than one hundred muscles. To signal the muscles to move, your brain does its own kind of "thinking," although you're not aware of it as it happens.

The brain doesn't use words to communicate with the muscles. It sends them electrical commands or signals, which travel through your nerves. When the signals get to your muscles, they cause a shift in the chemical balance inside the muscle cells. That change makes the muscle contract, or squeeze. And off you go.

All the squeezing and relaxing involved in movement is hard work, and your muscles need a supply of food and oxygen to give them the energy to do it.

The fuel is carried in your blood. When you exercise—say, during a brisk walk on a winter afternoon—your body has to keep the supply of fuel coming. To accomplish this, you breathe more quickly and take deeper breaths. That brings in more oxygen. Your heart starts beating faster, too, pumping more blood to deliver the oxygen to all your hardworking cells.

As your muscles work, they release energy in the form of heat, which warms you up. That's why you get home from a brisk walk feeling warm and relaxed all over.

Your body gets the most benefit from walking if you stretch gently before you start out, and gradually increase the pace of your stride until you're walking at a smooth, fairly fast pace. Swing your arms and enjoy your walk. Your brain will take care of putting one foot in front of the other.

What would happen if I didn't have thumbs?

It's easy to forget about your thumbs. Jamie, a fourth-grader, hadn't ever thought about his until he hurt one of them. He was

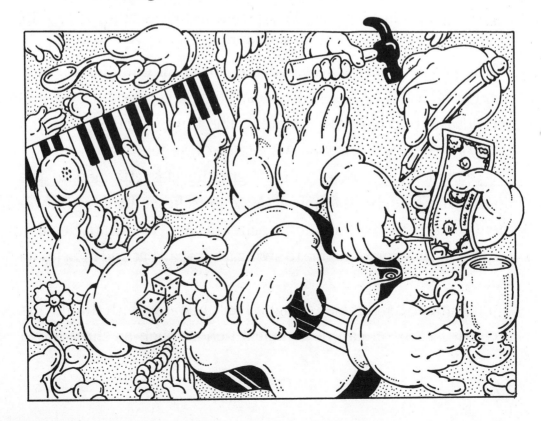

playing shortstop in a softball game, and as he tried to catch a ball, he used the hand without the mitt. He made the catch—but he also cracked the bone in his thumb.

Jamie's parents took him to the emergency room, where he had his hand put in a cast. "You won't be able to play softball for a while," his doctor told him.

At home, Jamie discovered that playing ball wasn't the only thing he wouldn't be able to do while his thumb was taped up. He couldn't do dishes, but that didn't bother him much. He couldn't tie the laces on his sneakers. He couldn't practice the piano. And he couldn't write or draw, because he's right-handed and his right thumb was the one he broke.

As Jamie found out, human beings have a particularly useful kind of thumb. It's called *opposable,* which means that we can move it separately from our fingers, and move it across our palms to meet each fingertip. Only human beings, monkeys, and apes have this kind of thumb.

Our opposable thumbs make our hands into amazingly useful tools. We can use them to do precise work such as painting a picture or mending a watch. The thumb also gives us a strong grip, so we can do things such as throw baseballs with one hand.

The human hand is a complicated piece of equipment. Each hand contains twenty-seven bones. They're connected by joints that let the bones move separately. The bumpy knuckles on the back of the hand show where some of these joints are.

A complex network of thirty-eight muscles attached to the bones causes the hand to move. Some muscles control fine movements—such as the touch of a piano player. Other muscles can grip hard, allowing someone to swing a baseball bat and hit a home run.

The human hand is also designed for grasping. With thumb and fingertip, a person can do a delicate chore such as threading a needle. This kind of hold is called a *precision grip*. Using another kind of grip, a *power grip*—with fingers and thumb curled around an object that's resting on the palm—gives extra hold for tough jobs such as hammering.

There's an experiment you can try to find out just how useful your thumbs are. Read more about it in the activity section on page 131.

I think people's feet are funny-looking. Why do they look that way?

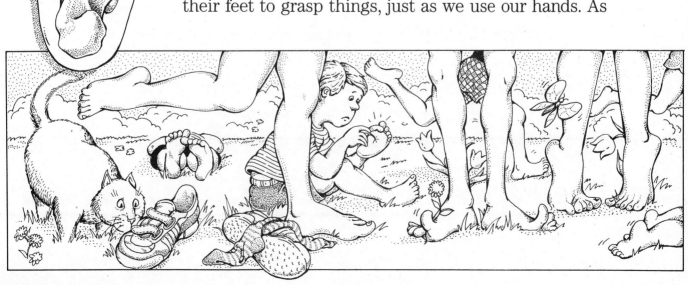

Feel your feet with your hands. You'll find a complicated set of bones—twenty-six separate bones in each foot. Since the average human skeleton contains about 206 bones, you can see that each foot contains about one-eighth of all the bones in your body.

Your feet are movable because thirty-three joints in each one allow you to change the position of the bones. Flexible bands of tissue stretched between the bones hold all this complicated machinery together. These bands are called ligaments. Each one of your feet has one hundred ligaments.

A long, long time ago, human beings' ancestors used their feet to grasp things, just as we use our hands. As time went on, these apelike human ancestors started to walk upright. The bones designed for grasping stayed the same. But the muscles around them changed.

The muscles in your feet aren't as complicated as those in your hands, although they work in similar ways. The feet are flexible, but not as much as the hands. You might be able to hold a pencil with your toes, but you'd have a hard time writing a letter that way—although some people have trained themselves to do that.

You might think your baby toe isn't good for much, but it helps you keep your balance. Your big toe is there to help you walk. Each time you take a step, it's like losing your balance, falling forward, and then catching yourself with your foot. When you push your weight forward, you push off with your big toe. It has a bigger, thicker bone than the other toes.

The skin on your feet is designed to take a lot of pressure from standing and walking. The bottoms of your feet have thicker skin than the rest of your body does. Your toenails provide protection, too. Imagine what it would be like to wear shoes if you didn't have any toenails.

But all the complicated stuff in your feet can cause trouble. Some experts say that foot problems are the most common ailment Americans have—after colds and tooth decay. That's not very surprising when you think about the job your feet have to do.

All your life, your feet carry you around. They must balance and support your entire body. Your feet cushion your weight when you run or jump—often on hard pavement, which doesn't give the way dirt or sand does when you land on it. One day's worth of walking puts a lot of weight on your feet—an amount equal to a few hundred tons by the time you finally go to bed at night!

What's the use of having hair and fingernails?

Have you ever seen a cat when it's outdoors in the winter? It fluffs up its fur into a thick coat to protect itself from the cold. When you feel chilly and get goose bumps, your hair stands up, too. But your "coat" isn't nearly as snuggly and warm as the one the cat wears.

You and that cat have something in common. You are both members of a group of animals called *mammals*. All mammals—from huge whales to tiny mice—have hair. Whales have only a few bristles around their mouths. But most other mammals are almost completely covered with hair.

Take a close look at your arms, legs, and face. You'll notice that tiny, short hairs cover your skin. Human beings have hair almost everywhere but the soles of the feet, the palms of the hands, and the lips. Some people have a lot of hair; others only have a little.

The hair on your head keeps you warm in the

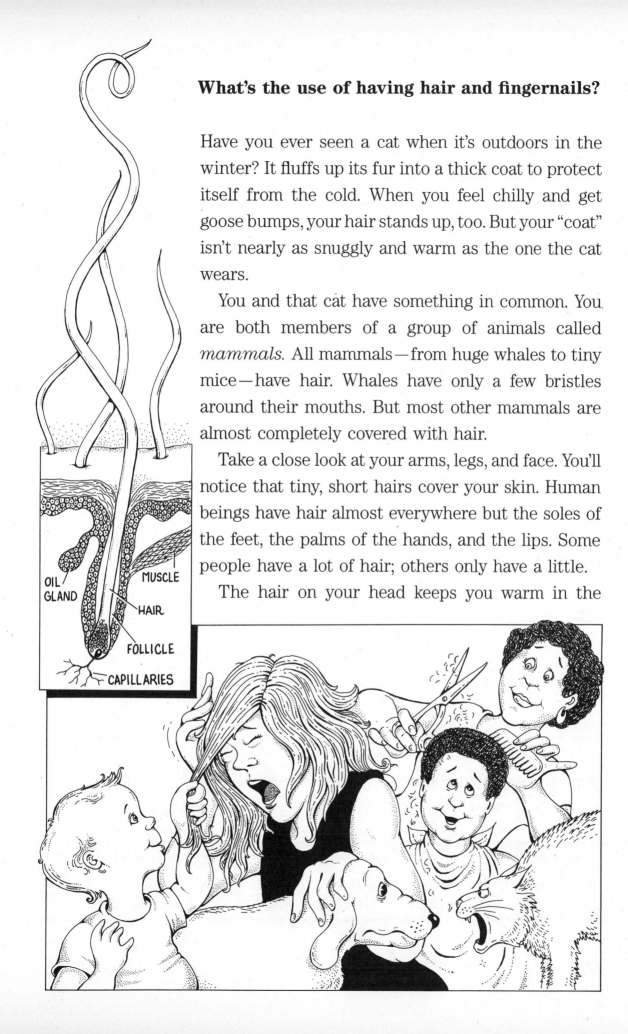

OIL GLAND

MUSCLE

HAIR

FOLLICLE

CAPILLARIES

winter. In the summer, hair shields your scalp from the sun.

Your eyebrows catch sweat and prevent it from running into your eyes when you exercise. They also act as natural sun visors by cutting down on the amount of light that glares into your eyes on a sunny day.

Your eyelashes keep bits of dust and bugs from getting into your eyes. Eyelashes are also very sensitive. If something touches them, they send nerve signals that alert your eyes to danger. Your eyelids blink shut.

Have you ever wondered why it doesn't hurt to get your hair cut, but it does hurt to get your hair pulled? The shaft of each hair—the part you can see—is made up of dead cells. When scissors cut through them, they don't send a pain message to the brain. But the roots of your hair are alive. When someone pulls on your hair, the roots flash out a pain message and you say "Ouch!"

A tough material called *keratin* forms your hair. Each hair grows as new cells form at its root. The cells push outward, building a shaft. Eventually, the hair dies and falls out. But a new hair grows in to replace it.

Keratin also forms your tough fingernails and toenails. Animals' claws are made of keratin, too. So are horses' hooves. Your nails aren't as tough as hooves, but they do protect the ends of your fingers and toes. The part you can see is made of dead cells, so it doesn't hurt to clip your nails—just as it doesn't hurt to cut your hair.

When people feel horrified or scared they sometimes say, "It made my hair stand on end!" Have you ever felt that way? Here's how it happens: Each hair on your body comes equipped with a tiny muscle that can make it stick upright. This muscle gets a message from your nerves when you are especially scared, angry, or excited. Similar nerve signals flash to the muscles when you feel cold.

Remember the fluffy cat in the cold? The hairs that form its coat have muscles, too. Cats, dogs, and most other mammals also have these muscles. When dogs growl at each other, their muscles make the hairs on the backs of their necks stand on end. Some wild animals fluff up their coats this way to look larger and fiercer when they meet an enemy.

When you feel scared or threatened, and your hair stands on end, your body is responding much as an animal's does—but instead of looking fierce, you look bumpy. Maybe that's why people use their hair mainly as decoration nowadays, instead of depending on it to scare away enemies.

Why do I shiver when I'm out in cold weather?

On a chilly, windy morning in January you bundle up well before you leave the house to walk to school. But by the time you get there, your body is shivering and your teeth are chattering. Brrrr!

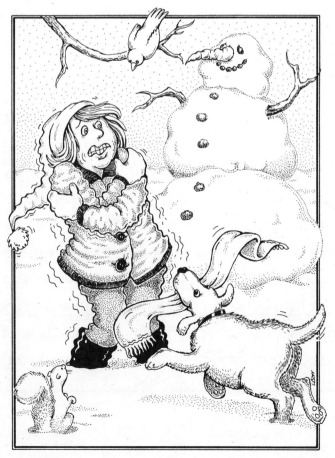

There's nothing wrong with you. In fact, your body is doing you a favor by shaking and shivering like a leaf in the wind. You may feel cold, but the movement in your muscles is actually keeping you warm.

As a human being, you're a warm-blooded animal. One of the things the millions and millions of cells in your body do is to use the food you eat to produce heat. When you're well, and in a comfortable environment, the temperature inside your body stays about the same all the time.

Look closely at the skin on your face. You'll see that it's covered with tiny holes called *pores*. Pores cover the rest of your body, too. When you feel hot, these pores open up. Sweat pours out of them. As the sweat dries, your body cools off. But during the winter your pores close up tight, shutting warmth inside. It's almost like shutting your bedroom window on a freezing night.

Your skin covers your body like a perfectly fitted glove. The outer layer—the part you see—is called the *epidermis*. Under that layer is another part of the skin called the *dermis*. Your dermis contains blood vessels and nerve cells. The nerves in your dermis make you very sensitive. They allow you to feel the difference between hot and cold.

When your nerves sense the cold, they carry a message to a part of your brain called the *hypothalamus*. The hypothalamus keeps track of the temperature of your blood. When your blood starts to cool, the hypothalamus goes into action. It sends signals racing through your body. Your blood vessels tighten. Less blood goes to the surface of your body, where it can lose heat quickly. Your skin cools off—but the important parts of you inside stay warm.

When your skin gets cold—like when you've been outside sledding for an hour or so—the hypothalamus sends another kind of message to your muscles. They begin to move, and you warm up by shivering and shaking. Your muscles are squeezing together and

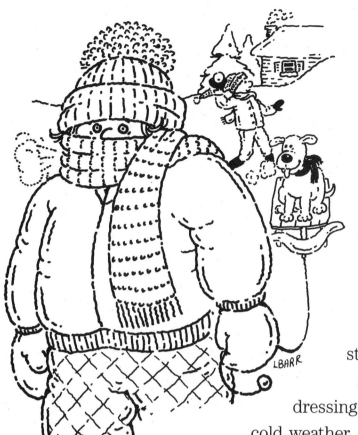

then relaxing again. They do it very quickly. As the muscles squeeze and relax, their cells produce extra heat. That keeps your body surface warm. You don't have to think about how cold you feel to get those signals from the hypothalamus going. Your body does the thinking for you. That kind of automatic response is called a *reflex*.

Your body has to work hard to stay warm when the air around it is very cold. You can help by dressing warmly when you go outside in cold weather, and remembering to wear a hat.

Can my skin really freeze if I stay out in the cold too long?

Yes, it can. You can be so cold that it hurts! Most of the time, you can warm up quickly after playing outside. But there are times when getting too cold can be dangerous.

A condition called *frostbite* occurs when skin and the tissue underneath it freeze. Most of the time, your body can keep itself warm enough to prevent this. But at very low temperatures, your system just can't send enough blood to the surface of the skin to keep it warm.

Your normal body temperature is about 98.6 degrees Fahrenheit. At that temperature, your inner organs—your heart, lungs, kidneys, liver, and so on—all work well. In very cold conditions, your body automatically cuts down on the flow of blood to your extremities—parts of your body far from the heart, such as your hands, feet, and face. That explains why your hands and feet and your ears and the tip of your nose are the first things to get cold when you spend a long time outside in the winter.

By cutting down on blood flow to the extremities and skin, your body conserves, or saves, heat for the important organs inside. The blood stays warm because it's staying away from the cold air outside.

Most cases of frostbite occur when the air outside is 20 degrees Fahrenheit or lower. But it can happen on warmer days if the wind is blowing too hard. Check the weather conditions when you're getting ready to go outside.

If the temperature of the body's extremities falls below about 25 degrees, frostbite sets in. The moisture in the skin and tissues literally freezes solid like an ice cube. The ice crystals that form can harm blood vessels and cells.

But even when it's below 20 degrees, you can't just stay inside all day and wait for spring. You need to do such things as standing at the school bus stop or walking to the store. There are some things you can do to avoid frostbite while you're out there.

ALWAYS WEAR A HAT. It's true that you lose a lot of heat through the top of your head. A hat warms the blood moving through your head, and helps the body keep itself warm.

DRESS WARMLY. Layers of loose clothing trap warm air around your body. Cotton socks worn under wool socks help keep the feet warm and dry. Mittens are warmer than gloves because the fingers keep each other warm. Tight gloves can cut off blood circulation in the fingers.

DON'T GET WET. As water on the skin evaporates, it cools the blood below the surface of the skin—just the opposite of what you want.

COVER UP BARE SKIN. If it's very cold and windy, putting a scarf across your nose and cheeks will protect them.

IF YOU'RE SO COLD THAT IT HURTS, GET INSIDE. The pain is your body's warning signal.

If you start to feel numb, it's even more important to get inside fast. As frostbite sets in, the area feels tingly at first. Then it hurts. Then—as nerves freeze—it gets numb.

How can you recognize frostbite? The frostbitten part of the body will feel hard and either numb or tingly. The area will look white, gray, or bluish white because blood flow has been cut off. Usually, the ears, nose, cheeks, fingers, and toes are the first areas of the body to get frostbitten.

Injuries from the cold can often be seen before the victim feels them. So in really cold weather it's important to play outdoors with a buddy instead of alone.

My sunburn is killing me. Why did my skin get burned?

You had a wonderful day at the beach. You built a sand castle, played volleyball, and finally figured out how to stand up on a surfboard. Now you're getting ready to go to sleep—but there's a problem. Your skin is so sore that you can't find a comfortable position in which to lie down. It's also red, and it feels hot to the touch.

You have a bad sunburn.

People need to absorb a certain amount of sunlight for good health. The light helps your body produce vitamins needed to

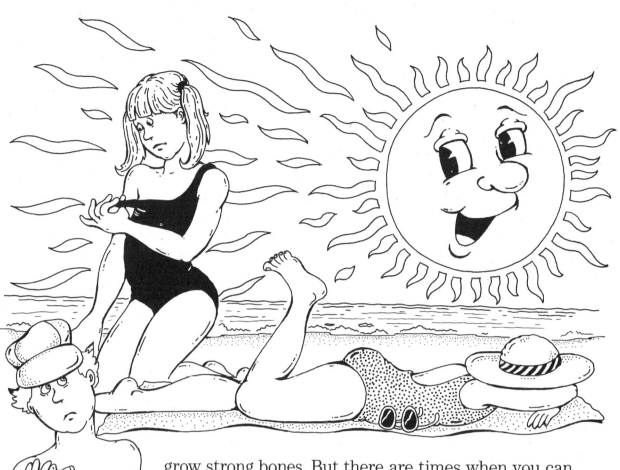

grow strong bones. But there are times when you can get too much of a good thing—such as after a long day at the beach without sunscreen or protective clothing.

Sunlight contains invisible rays called *ultraviolet light.* These are the rays that burn your skin. If you've ever gotten too much sun you know that it really hurts. You may feel feverish and sick. And even after you feel better, you usually have to put up with having the top layer of your skin peel off. That may be fine if you're a snake—but it's not much fun for a person.

When you get a sunburn, the blood vessels near your skin swell up. This is your body's way of bringing extra blood to the surface to help you heal. But in the meantime, you look and feel pretty uncomfortable.

Getting sunburned can have even more serious con-

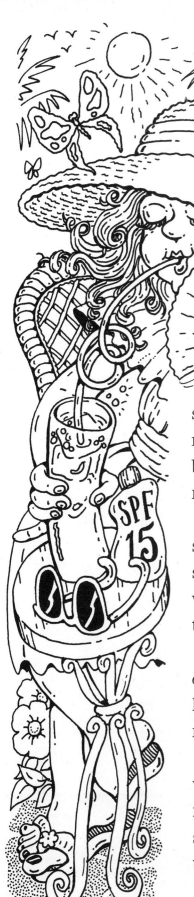

sequences than that, however. Doctors have found that years of letting too much ultraviolet light soak into the skin makes the skin dry out and lose its ability to stretch. Someone who gets too much sun early in life can end up with skin that looks wrinkled and saggy before he or she is old.

Skin cancer, a serious disease, can also be caused by too much sun. Scientific studies show that people in the United States are getting more skin cancer now than they used to. Many scientists believe that's because so many Americans spend the summer soaking up sun.

Your body has a built-in defense system against the sun's harmful ultraviolet rays called *melanin*. It's the substance that makes your skin the color it is. Everyone—whether white, black, yellow, red, or brown—has melanin to color the skin.

Melanin is produced by special cells called *melanocytes*. If you are dark-skinned, your melanocytes make a lot of melanin. If you are light-skinned, they don't make as much.

When people go out in the sun, their melanocytes start working overtime. The cells start producing more melanin than usual. The melanin protects the skin, because it soaks up harmful ultraviolet rays before they can get through the skin and damage delicate tissues. This hap-

23

pens whether you are light-skinned or dark-skinned; it just happens in different amounts. Whether you are light- or dark-skinned, too much sun can cause changes in your cells that may eventually lead to skin cancer. Your melanin just can't provide all the protection you need.

That's why dermatologists—doctors who take care of the skin—recommend that people use protection when they go out in the hot summer sun. There are three basic rules:

AVOID THE SUN BETWEEN TEN IN THE MORNING AND TWO IN THE AFTERNOON. That's when the ultraviolet rays are at their strongest.

WEAR A HAT. It will protect your head and face when you do go out in strong sun.

USE A SUNSCREEN. The cream will protect your skin from harmful ultraviolet rays. Ask your parents to help you choose the best one for your skin type. Before going outside, put the sunscreen on all the parts of your skin that will be in the sun. That means the tips of your feet, the tips of your ears, and the part in your hair. A sunburned scalp can really hurt! Always put sunscreen on again after you go swimming. And don't be fooled by a cloudy day. The harmful rays of the sun can get through a cloud cover and burn you just as badly as they would on a sunny day.

If you follow these simple rules next time you go out in the sun, you'll be taking good care of your skin for future use.

Why do I blush when I get embarrassed? It's so embarrassing!

Let's say you drop a full tray of food right in the middle of the lunchroom. When something like that happens, you may feel your face flaming with a bright red blush. Your heart pounds. Your palms feel sweaty. You want to leap up and run away.

Embarrassment can be a very powerful feeling. When you're experiencing it, it seems to block out everything else for a few seconds. It's an emotion strong enough to affect your body.

When you feel a strong emotion, your body switches on two tiny little organs called the *adrenal glands*. The adrenal glands sit like little caps on top of each one of your kidneys. These small glands give off chemicals called *hormones*. The adrenal glands make two kinds of hormones: *adrenaline* and *noradrenaline*. These two substances increase your heart rate, raise your blood pressure, and make you produce more sweat. Your body automatically sends more blood to your muscles and brain. As the chemicals rush through your bloodstream they can also make you feel kind of shaky.

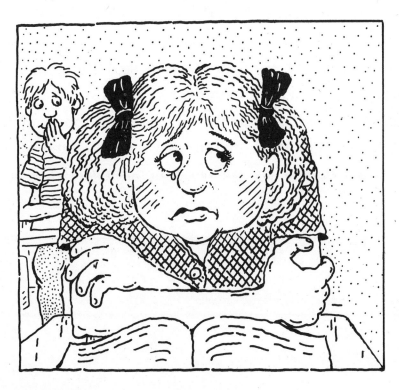

When your heart rate and blood pressure go up, more blood than usual reaches the surface of your skin. If you're fair—or very light-skinned—the extra blood pulsing through small veins near the surface of the skin shows clearly through the paper-thin outer layer called the epidermis. But dark-skinned people blush too. It's just not so obvious.

As the rush of hormones fades, the blush fades, too. The heartbeat slows down to a normal rate, and the "crisis" is over.

It may seem like an overreaction for the body to get so fired up over a simple case of embarrassment. But the *endocrine system*—the group of glands that regulate chemicals in the body—can't really tell whether the "crisis" started by a strong emotion is major or minor. The emotion happens, the system clicks on, and *bang!* your body is on the alert. This physical alarm system is like the "fight-or-flight" response in animals. An animal's nervous system clicks on to get it ready to run away or to turn and fight for survival on a moment's notice.

In human beings, the hormones released by the adrenal glands give the body the extra burst of energy and strength needed to respond to an emergency. During the short time that the hormones are coursing through the bloodstream, people can run faster, fight harder, or perform feats of strength that they couldn't usually manage. That moment could be something life-threatening, such as seeing a car running a red light toward your bicycle. Or it could be something emotional—such as having a fight with your best friend or receiving bad news about someone in your family. Or the "emergency" can be a humiliating incident at school.

I have a horrible wart. I look like a monster. I have moles on my skin, too. How did they get there?

Your skin is pretty tough. It has to be able to stand up to daily meetings with wind, weather, and germs. But sometimes germs do invade the skin. One of the things they cause is *warts*.

"Ugh," you say. "Warts are awful." It's true that warts aren't very pretty to look at—but they are pretty harmless. If you have ever had warts—and most kids have—you know that they tend to disappear as mysteriously as they appeared.

Some people think that warts appear from handling toads. Maybe that story got started because a toad's skin looks warty. But toads don't deserve their reputation, because warts are really caused by invisible germs called *viruses*.

Sometimes viruses get into cells on the outer surface of your skin and multiply. Eventually, a small, hard, lumpy bump appears.

Warts most commonly grow on the hands and feet. Some may appear on the face, as well as on the elbows and knees. Sometimes the ones that grow on the bottom of the feet can be painful. That's

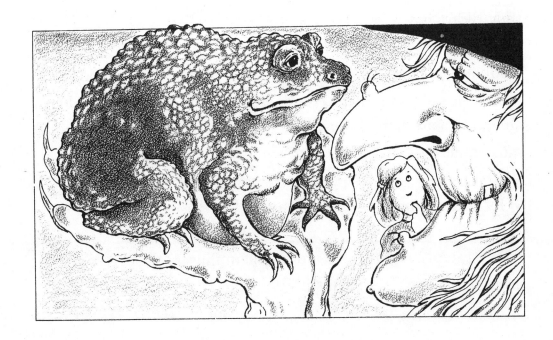

because the hard wart presses against the soft tissue in your foot as you walk.

When that happens, you may want to go to the doctor to see if the wart should be removed. It's not a very good idea to try to remove the wart with medicines you can buy in drugstores. They can burn the skin if you use them wrong.

Another kind of bump or mark also appears on the skin. Called a *mole*, it's a little patch of cells that has an extra amount of melanin, the coloring substance that makes your skin the shade it is. Melanin is concentrated in the mole.

When you were born, you probably didn't have any moles on your body. But as you grew, they began to show up. Doctors aren't absolutely sure why people have moles, but the location of the marks seems to be determined even before a baby is born.

More moles appear as a person becomes an adult. An average person has about fifty moles by the time he or she is grown up. Then they begin to fade away. If you live a very long life, most of your moles may completely disappear.

Many people think moles are attractive. They call them "beauty marks." Long ago, people used to glue false moles on their faces if they didn't have any natural ones.

Like warts, moles are basically harmless. But they can cause trouble if you pick at them or irritate them. If your moles get irritated, grow rapidly, or look different from usual, a doctor should look at them. It may be a good idea to have a troublesome mole removed.

Why did my baby teeth fall out?

It's a strange feeling to have your old familiar teeth start to wobble around in your mouth. But it's completely normal.

All human beings get two complete sets of teeth. The first set

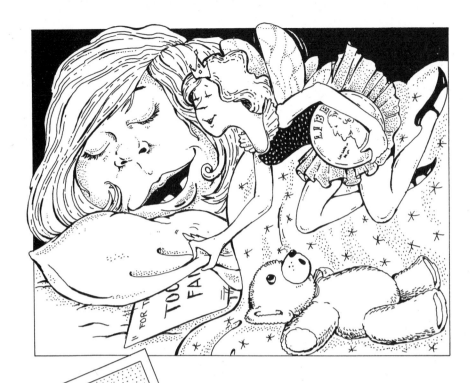

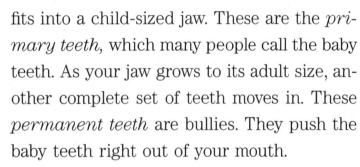

fits into a child-sized jaw. These are the *primary teeth,* which many people call the baby teeth. As your jaw grows to its adult size, another complete set of teeth moves in. These *permanent teeth* are bullies. They push the baby teeth right out of your mouth.

When you were born, you didn't have any teeth showing through your gums at all, but they had already started to grow in your jaw. They didn't begin to show in your mouth, though, until you were about six months old.

As you grew, you began to teethe, and your baby teeth slowly began to show through your gums. If there's a baby in your house, you know that teething can be unpleasant, because it makes the gums sore and tender. That makes the baby cranky and cry a lot.

Dentists call the small, white baby teeth

your *deciduous teeth*. The word *deciduous* means "falling." This means that the teeth aren't permanent; they will eventually fall out. Have you ever heard your science teacher talk about deciduous trees? Those are the trees with leaves that fall off in the autumn.

Teeth come in several different shapes. Take a look in the mirror. Your front teeth, designed for cutting, are called *incisors*. On either side of the incisors are your pointed *canine teeth*. The word canine means "doglike." Look at your pointed canines and compare them to a dog's teeth. Can you see the resemblance?

Two-pointed teeth called *bicuspids* come next. These teeth can tear and grind food. At the back of your mouth are the hard-working *molars*—broad, flat teeth that grind. They're the largest teeth in the mouth. You have eight molars in your first set of teeth. When all your permanent teeth come in, you have twelve.

It's important to take care of all of your teeth—primary and permanent. A healthy mouthful of primary teeth provides a good place for permanent teeth to grow, and helps them grow straight. If your primary teeth are full of cavities, the decay can spread to your permanent teeth.

The first permanent teeth to appear in your mouth are a set of four molars. Because most kids are about age six when this happens, dentists call the teeth the *six-year molars*. There's nothing to worry about if a six-year-old hasn't got those molars yet, though. A dental X ray will show that they're there in the jaw, just taking their time before they show up in the mouth.

As a child's baby teeth begin to fall out, the six-year molars come in handy. They can be used to chomp on food when some of the other teeth in the mouth are loose or missing.

The six-year molars also help to shape the lower part of the face. Once all four of these new permanent teeth are in place, they hold the jaws in position as the baby teeth gradually fall out and are replaced by larger permanent teeth. No wonder dentists often say that the six-year molars are the most important teeth in the mouth.

You probably already know that some of the baby teeth don't just fall out the way a leaf drifts from a tree. They may be loose and bothersome for weeks on end before they're ready to come out. It's okay to push at your loose tooth with your tongue. But if you push it too much, the gums around the tooth may get sore and red.

Each of your teeth has a root that anchors it in your jaw. As your permanent teeth force your baby teeth out, the baby teeth's roots slowly disappear. By the time baby teeth actually fall out, they may not have any root left at all. Then, a loose tooth will come out easily. Just a light tug, or even a slight push with the tongue, may do the trick.

Have you ever seen cartoons in which the characters pull out a loose tooth by tying a string to a doorknob and then slamming the door? Don't try it! You shouldn't try to force a tooth out until it's almost ready to fall out on its own.

I had a cavity in my tooth. The dentist gave me a filling. How can I avoid getting more cavities?

Cavities begin when tiny bacteria, or germs, in your mouth change the food you eat into a strong acid. The acid is so powerful it can literally eat holes in your teeth. When you brush your teeth, you remove the small bits of food that the bacteria in your mouth like to feed on. By taking away their meal, you keep the bacteria from producing acid.

If you go to bed without brushing your teeth, your teeth are likely to have a mossy feeling on them when you wake up the next morning. A substance called *plaque* formed on the teeth during the night. Plaque is a mixture of food, saliva, and bacteria. If

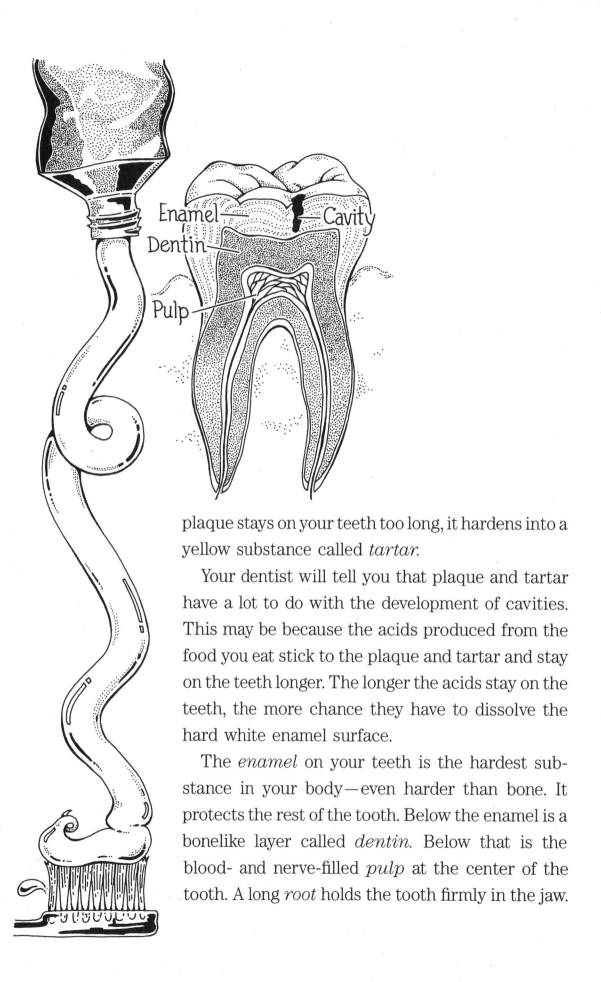

Enamel

Dentin

Pulp

Cavity

plaque stays on your teeth too long, it hardens into a yellow substance called *tartar.*

Your dentist will tell you that plaque and tartar have a lot to do with the development of cavities. This may be because the acids produced from the food you eat stick to the plaque and tartar and stay on the teeth longer. The longer the acids stay on the teeth, the more chance they have to dissolve the hard white enamel surface.

The *enamel* on your teeth is the hardest substance in your body—even harder than bone. It protects the rest of the tooth. Below the enamel is a bonelike layer called *dentin.* Below that is the blood- and nerve-filled *pulp* at the center of the tooth. A long *root* holds the tooth firmly in the jaw.

Tooth enamel is tough. But once it's damaged, it can't repair itself. When you get a scratch on your hand, the skin heals quickly. But when the enamel coating on the tooth gets a hole in it, the hole stays. Another word for the hole is a *cavity*. Once the hole is there, infection can spread inside your tooth, causing more decay.

When you get a cavity, your dentist removes the decayed part of the tooth with a high-speed drill. Then you get a filling made of a mixture of metals or plastic or even gold. Most kids never get cavities large enough to require gold fillings. But most kids do get cavities. By the time children in the United States reach age twelve, about 90 percent of them have some cavities.

The water you drink probably contains small amounts of chemicals called *fluorides*. The chemicals make the enamel on people's teeth harder and more resistant to acid. Fluorides help prevent tooth decay. You may also use a fluoride toothpaste or have fluoride treatments at the dentist to help prevent cavities. And as your dentist has probably told you, brushing and flossing after every meal, getting regular dental checkups, and avoiding too much sugar can help prevent cavities from forming.

2

THE INSIDE STORY

Many of the important jobs your body does—such as breathing, eating, and pumping blood—go on under the surface of your skin where you can't watch them happen. This chapter answers some questions about how the internal organs in your body work, and why the things they do are so important.

Does my heart really look like a valentine? How does my heart work?

On Valentine's Day you give your friends heart-shaped cards. But those cards don't really show what your heart looks like.

Your heart is a hollow muscle about the same size as your fist. It's shaped quite a bit like a fist, too. If you use your imagination, you might still think your heart looks something like a valentine.

Whether you're sound asleep or running the hundred-yard dash, your heart beats all the time.

When you put your hand on the upper left side of your chest,

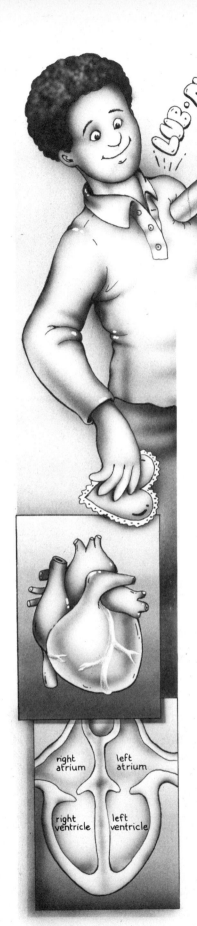

right atrium

left atrium

right ventricle

left ventricle

you can feel your heart beating. What you're feeling is the lower end of the heart, which tips toward the front of the body. Most of your heart is located in the center of your chest, protected by the bones that form your rib cage.

Your heart has a very important job. It pumps blood through your body to bring oxygen and food to your cells. You get the oxygen from the air you breathe. The oxygen keeps your cells—and you—alive.

Try imagining that your heart muscle is a box with four rooms inside it—two rooms on top, and two rooms on the bottom. The box is a kind of recycling center for your blood.

Blood coming back from its trip through the body enters the top room on the right. This blood has delivered all of its oxygen to the body. A door opens, and the blood moves into the bottom room on the right. From there, it flows through another door to the lungs.

While the blood is in the lungs, it picks up more oxygen.

35

As the oxygen-carrying blood leaves the lungs, it gathers in the top left room of the heart. Once the room is full, a door opens and the blood flows into the bottom room on the left side. From this room, the oxygen-carrying blood travels to the rest of the body to deliver its fresh load of oxygen.

Doctors call the heart and the network of vessels the *cardio-vascular system.* "Cardio" means heart, and "vascular" means veins and arteries.

Your heart beats about 100,000 times every day, even when you're asleep. How does it keep going?

Inside your heart is a small patch of cells that sends out electrical signals. These signals tell the heart muscle when to squeeze and pump the blood through its chambers—those four rooms you just read about. Doctors call the small patch of cells your *pace-maker.* Like your heart, it's on the job all the time.

From your heart, your blood moves through your body in a very complicated network of tubes called *blood vessels.* Your heart and blood vessels together make up your *circulatory system.* You have so many blood vessels to circulate your blood through the body that if they were all connected and laid out in a row, they would stretch for thousands of miles. In your body, they reach every bit of you, from your brain to the tips of your toes.

You can feel your blood moving if you put your fingers on one of the blood vessels located near the surface of your body. You can feel this pulse on the inside of your wrist. You can also feel it on either side of your neck, near your jaw line. You might also be able to feel it on your temples. Each little thump that you feel is the result of your heart pumping the blood along. You can monitor your heart's action by taking your pulse. Find out how on page 130.

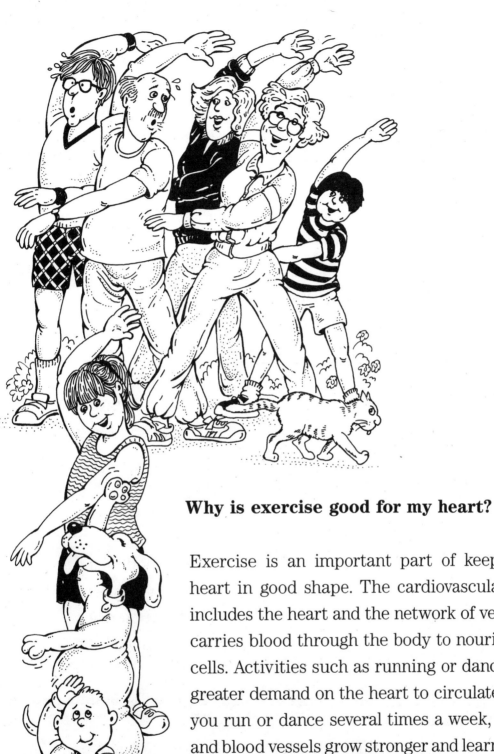

Why is exercise good for my heart?

Exercise is an important part of keeping your heart in good shape. The cardiovascular system includes the heart and the network of vessels that carries blood through the body to nourish all the cells. Activities such as running or dancing put a greater demand on the heart to circulate blood. If you run or dance several times a week, the heart and blood vessels grow stronger and learn to circulate blood without working as hard.

Let's say you take part in a relay race. To you, it's a game. But your body is doing a tough job. Your leg muscles work hard, burning up energy. Your heart muscle squeezes harder than usual to pump blood to the hard-working muscles. As you run, your heart will pump several times as much blood each minute as it does when you're resting.

When you keep up an activity such as running, swimming, fast walking, or biking for several minutes at a stretch, you're doing *aerobic* exercise. Aerobic means "using oxygen." This kind of activity requires deep breathing to bring in extra oxygen for hardworking muscles to use as fuel. Regular aerobic exercise helps keep you fit and strengthens your heart.

Dr. William Strong, a heart specialist, works with children at the University of Georgia to find out how to help them avoid heart trouble later in life. He emphasizes the importance of a good diet and plenty of exercise. He says that making these practices a regular part of your life is important no matter how old you are. But if you're young, healthy heart habits give you a head start at avoiding problems such as high blood pressure and certain kinds of heart disease.

Dr. Strong says that kids should exercise regularly by taking an active part in school physical education programs. Stay active during vacation time, too.

But exercise alone isn't enough. "Kids should eat a good mixed diet that is nutritionally sound," Dr. Strong adds. That doesn't mean you have to give up every single cookie or French fry forever, though. Instead, Dr. Strong says, "Use moderation." That means be sensible about what you eat and don't overdo it.

"The most important thing of all," Dr. Strong adds, "is never, ever pick up a cigarette."

Sometimes an afternoon TV show may sound like more fun than playing kick ball with the kids in the neighborhood. If you feel that way, think again. Remember your heart has to pump a total of 8,000 gallons of blood 12,000 miles through your body every day. You can make its job easier by getting regular exercise.

Why did my grandma have to change her diet after her heart attack? She's supposed to cut back on cholesterol.

Sometimes a heart attack is like a warning. The person who had the attack has another chance. Your grandmother's new eating habits will help her live a longer and healthier life. Part of watching her diet means cutting back on foods with a lot of *cholesterol* in them.

Cholesterol is a fatty material. The body uses it in many different chemical processes. But when too much cholesterol moves through the body in the blood, it can cause trouble.

Medical researchers have found that in some people, cholesterol can gum up the cardiovascular system. Cholesterol leaves deposits on the inside of blood vessels, making them narrower than normal. This narrowing, or blockage, can cause chest pain. If the blockage

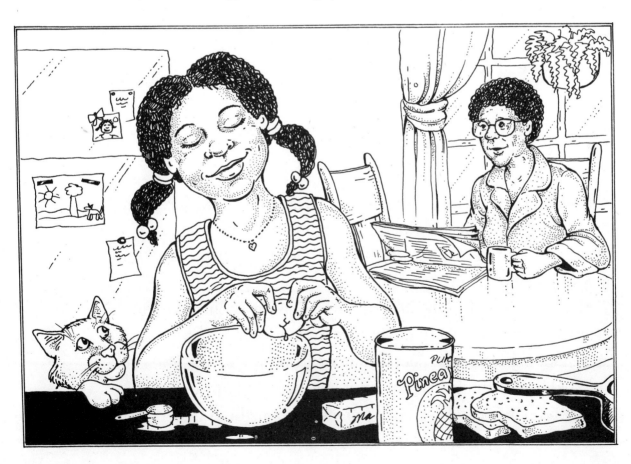

gets serious enough, it can interfere with the flow of blood and oxygen in the heart itself, leading to a heart attack.

Egg yolks and organ meats such as liver are very high in cholesterol. So your grandmother has probably had to give up her favorite breakfast of two fried eggs and a couple of sausages. A breakfast of cereal, fruit, and low-fat milk is healthier for her heart.

Many experts think that learning to avoid food that can cause cardiovascular problems many years later is a good idea. To keep the heart healthy, it's important to know the rules of good nutrition. The science of nutrition concerns the foods we eat and how our bodies use them. Nutritionists recommend that we eat a variety of servings from the four main food groups every day. The groups are:

- Poultry and lean meats
- Milk and milk products
- Bread and cereals
- Fruits and vegetables

Why shouldn't I smoke?

Do you know the story of Tom Sawyer? If so, you probably remember that he and his friend Huckleberry Finn tried out smoking one afternoon. Puffing on pipes made them feel pretty grown up—but it also made them pretty sick.

Mark Twain wrote the story of Tom Sawyer about a hundred years ago. Since then, scientists have learned a lot about just how sick smoking can make people—in fact, that it can kill. Even so, some kids still think that smoking is a cool thing to do.

To find out why you shouldn't smoke, you need to understand

how your *respiratory system*—the part of you that does your breathing—works. Let's follow a breath as it moves through your lungs and back out again.

First the air enters your body through your nose and mouth. Hairs inside your nostrils catch particles of dirt that may be in the air. The lining of your nose is called *mucous membrane,* which secretes a wet, sticky substance called *mucus.* It captures some of the pollution, germs, and dust in the air and keeps them from going down into your lungs.

Your respiratory system, like your nose, is coated with a sticky mucous lining. In it, tiny hairlike bumps called *cilia* constantly sway back and forth. The cilia are so small that they can only be seen through a microscope. You have millions of them lining your respiratory tract.

The cilia's job is to sweep away dirt and germs. They do this by waving back and forth about twelve times per second. They sweep the bad things toward your mouth and nose, where they can be disposed of. When you cough or sneeze, you get rid of these unwelcome particles.

From your mouth and nose, the breath of air you inhaled, which contains oxygen, moves on to your *lungs.* The air swooshes into your throat and down your windpipe, or *trachea.* From there, the breath flows into a system of tubes called the *bronchial tree.* The bronchial tree fills your lungs, two football-size organs inside your chest. Put your hands on your chest and take a few deep breaths. You'll feel your lungs getting bigger and smaller as you breathe in and out.

Wait a minute—a tree inside your lungs?

Your bronchial tree isn't a real tree, of course. It's a branching system of passages that looks like an upside-down tree without any leaves. Like branches and twigs, the air passages of your bronchial tree gradually get smaller and smaller. At the tips of the smallest parts are small clusters of sacs called *alveoli*. They have a very important job to do.

The oxygen in the air you breathe enters your blood through the alveoli. Parts of your blood called *red blood cells* soak up the oxygen. Then your heart pumps the oxygen-rich blood through your body. That oxygen keeps you alive.

When your red cells pick up oxygen at the alveoli, they leave behind another gas called *carbon dioxide*. Carbon dioxide is the waste product left over after your cells use up oxygen. This harmful gas leaves the body when you breathe out, or exhale.

So why shouldn't you mix tobacco smoke in with the air you breathe? There are lots of reasons.

Tobacco smoke contains many harmful things. It has a chemical called *nicotine* in it. When nicotine enters your body it makes your blood vessels get smaller. Then your heart has to work harder to pump blood through them.

Tars in cigarette smoke coat the inside of your nice pink lungs, turning them brown. Substances in the cigarette smoke also cause lung cancer, a very serious disease that kills many people every year. Smoking is the leading cause of this deadly cancer.

Tobacco smoke also contains *carbon monoxide*. When this gas reaches your alveoli, it passes into your red blood cells. This prevents them from picking up their load of oxygen—so a smaller amount of this important gas reaches your cells.

42

Cigarette smoke is also very hot. It rushes into your lungs fast, and burns the sensitive lining of your bronchial tree.

Remember those cilia that work so hard to sweep away harmful particles in the air you breathe? Just one cigarette slows the action of the cilia. If someone smokes for a long time, the cilia get paralyzed. Very heavy smoking can even destroy the cilia. When cilia stop working well, more germs enter the lungs.

The American Lung Association reports that a million American teenagers start smoking every year. The Lung Association's advice to kids is: *Don't Start.* If you never start, your respiratory system will keep you breathing easy for a long, long time.

Why do I need to eat so much? I play a lot of soccer, and it seems like I'm starving all the time.

Food is the fuel that keeps the human body going. It provides the energy we need to do everything from sleeping to solving a math

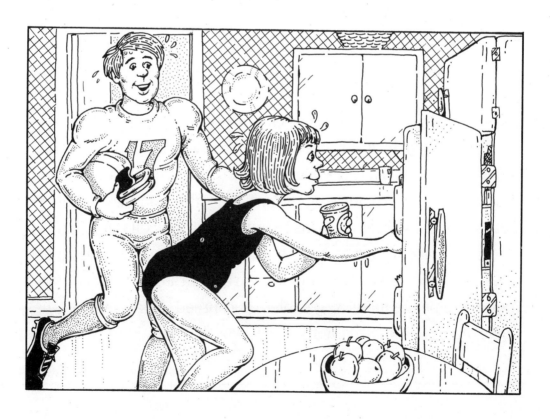

problem. Nutritionists measure the energy we get from our food in units called *calories*.

During our daily activities we burn up the calories contained in the food we've eaten. Just staying alive—breathing and keeping the heart beating and the blood moving—takes energy.

An average adult needs between 1,300 and 1,600 calories a day. Growing kids aged seven to ten need an average of about 2,400 calories. Boys aged eleven to fourteen need an average of 2,700 calories, while girls that age need 2,200. It's important to remember that these numbers are averages only. You may need fewer or more calories, depending on how big you are and how much exercise you get. If you wonder about your own individual needs, ask your doctor.

Young athletes, for example, may need to add more calories to meet the demands of their sport. Kids who spend hours practicing strenuous activities such as soccer or gymnastics use up more calories than less athletic kids do. The athletes have to eat more to make up the difference. Extremely athletic kids in the seven-to-ten age group might need as many as 3,000 to 4,000 calories a day. Some of the calories fuel their athletic activity. The rest give the energy needed for growth. Getting those calories isn't usually a problem, though. Young athletes usually have huge appetites!

A good way to get the extra calories you may need if you're athletic is to increase the amount of *carbohydrates* in your diet. Carbohydrates provide energy and help the body soak up *proteins*. The body uses proteins to build cells, the cells that make up everything from your hair and toenails to your muscles and blood.

Among the foods that provide carbohydrates are fruits, corn, potatoes, pasta, many vegetables, and bread. Meat, poultry, fish, eggs, and cheese are among the foods that provide protein.

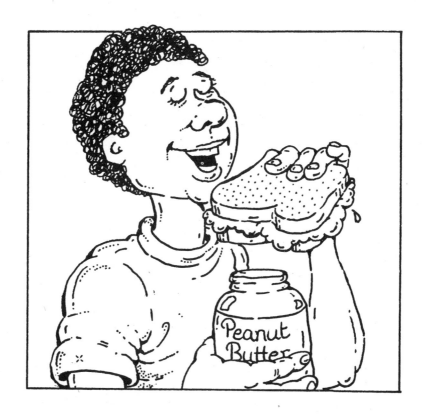

What happens to my food after I swallow it?

Your *digestive system* is in charge of breaking down the food you eat into parts small enough for the cells in your body to use for fuel. The process actually starts before you even swallow your first bite.

Think about Thanksgiving. When you walk into a house where a turkey has been roasting for hours, you smell a delicious aroma. When you smell it, and see the brown turkey resting on its platter, your body immediately goes to work. The sight and smell of the food makes special glands in your mouth produce *saliva,* or spit. That's when you say, "The food looks so good my mouth is watering."

Your saliva will come in handy when you start eating the turkey, stuffing, potatoes, and vegetables on your plate. When you take your first bite, *digestion* begins.

Before your body can use it, your bite of turkey has to be chewed up. Your teeth are specially designed to do this. Some of them are sharp and pointed for cutting; others are designed for grinding. As you chew, your saliva mixes with the food. It makes the food moist and slippery so that it will move down your throat comfortably. At the same time, *enzymes* found in the saliva start changing the bite of turkey, breaking it down into substances your body can absorb.

The next step is swallowing. Your *tongue,* which is very muscular, squeezes the food into a wad and pushes it toward the back of your throat. From there it passes into the *esophagus.* The food doesn't fall into the esophagus like a penny into a wishing well, though. Strong muscles squeeze it down toward your *stomach.*

You don't need to think about the muscles in your esophagus to move them; they work automatically. They're powerful enough to move food to your stomach even if you're standing on your head.

In your stomach, your bite of turkey gets a bath in strong liquids called *digestive juices.* Your stomach's muscular walls churn these juices with the food, mixing it up into a creamy liquid. At this point, the food you swallowed doesn't look much like turkey anymore. But it's almost ready to start being useful to your cells.

The next stop on the digestive tract is your *small intestine.* This twisting and turning tube isn't actually small at all. If you stretched it out, it would be several times taller than you are. It gets its name from the small opening between it and your stomach. The most important part of digestion takes place in the small intestine.

A thick lining of tiny finger-shaped bumps covers the inside of the small intestine, forming a shaggy lining. You have about 5 million of these bumps, which are called *villi.* As the churned-up food moves through the small intestine, the villi soak up the useful parts and transfer them into your blood. The blood then delivers the food to every cell in your body.

But not all of the food you eat can be used. Some of it passes on into the *large intestine.* The large intestine is actually shorter than the small intestine—it's only about 5 feet long—but it has a larger opening than the small intestine does. This large opening gives it its name.

The walls of the large intestine soak up water from your food and return it to the body. The solid, useless parts of your food pass out of your large intestine when you go to the bathroom.

Some parts of the digestion process are fast. You chew your food for less than a minute, and the esophagus moves it to the stomach in a few seconds more. The stomach churns your meal for several hours before it turns it over to your small intestine, where it may take as long as eight hours getting through. A meal takes between twelve and fifteen hours to go through the whole digestive system. So if you eat your Thanksgiving turkey in the late afternoon or early evening, it delivers fuel to your cells around the time you get out of bed on Friday morning.

A Thanksgiving meal provides very useful fuel. The protein in the turkey helps build cells. Protein forms about three-fourths of the solid parts of you, such as skin, hair, bones, and muscles.

The carbohydrates in the potatoes and bread you eat with your turkey provide energy to keep your body moving.

Calcium, a mineral in the milk you drink, helps keep your bones and teeth strong.

Your vegetables provide vitamins to keep your body chemistry balanced, and bulk to keep your digestive system working smoothly.

And if you finish off your Thanksgiving feast with a piece of pumpkin pie, you get a rich helping of vitamin A. Orange vegetables such as squash and pumpkin contain *carotene,* a substance that gives them their bright color. In your body, carotene changes to Vitamin A. Vitamin A helps your eyes see at night, and also helps keep your skin and bones in good shape.

When you wake up the day after Thanksgiving full of health and energy, you'll have one more thing to be thankful for—the good job your digestive system did with your meal.

Why does my stomach growl when I'm hungry?

It's near the end of math class. Everyone's working on a few problems. The room is quiet, except for the sound of pencils scratching across paper. You've already finished, and as you wait for your teacher to collect the paper you start thinking about the chicken sandwich that's in your lunch box. You can imagine taking the first bite ...

Suddenly you hear a strange sound: GRRRRRRRRRRRRRR. It's coming from your stomach. How embarrassing!

Everyone's stomach growls now and then. In fact, stomach-growling has a fancy scientific name. Next time your stomach starts to growl, tell your giggling friend that it's nothing to worry about, you just have *borborygmi.*

Borborygmi may make you blush when it happens in a quiet place, but the noise is a normal event. It's a sign that your stomach is doing its job—creating digestive juices and churning them around inside. The muscular walls of your stomach whoosh the juices around like a washing machine churning water, and the sounds begin. When you feel the churnings, you know that you're hungry.

After a meal, your stomach and the rest of your digestive system continue to make noises. You can hear them if you put your ear

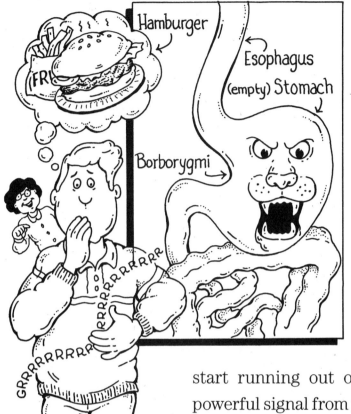

Hamburger

Esophagus

(empty) Stomach

Borborygmi

GRRRRRRRRRRRRRRRRRRR

against a friend's belly. Those gurgling noises are the sounds of digestion.

If you play soccer outside on a cold day, you're likely to feel very hungry afterward. You may even run into the kitchen at home yelling, "I'm starving." That's an exaggeration, of course. It takes a lot longer than the length of a soccer game for the human body to really start running out of fuel. But you are getting a powerful signal from your body that says: "Feed me!"

Then, after you gobble up a snack, you feel satisfied. If someone offers you a second helping you may say, "No, thanks, I'm stuffed." Even if there's a piece of your favorite kind of pie in front of you, you can't imagine eating it.

You feel full because you are full, of course. Your stomach—a muscular, pear-shaped bag located right between your ribs above your belly button—has something to work on. Nerve endings in your stomach send signals to your brain saying, "Enough."

The feeling you call hunger is pretty complicated. It's not just a matter of emptying your stomach and filling it up again at regular times. Your brain plays a role in your eating patterns, too.

After your stomach has finished its job and sent the food along to the next stage in the digestion process, you still won't feel hungry for a while. That's because the part of your brain that controls your appetite knows that your body still has enough fuel to keep it working for some time.

The device that keeps track of how warm your house is is called a thermostat. Scientists call the part of the brain that controls eating behavior your *appestat*. They are still trying to figure out exactly how the appestat decides when to tell you to eat or to stop eating. They know that the appestat is located in a part of your brain called the *hypothalamus*. This walnut-size section of your brain is also in charge of such vital things as your body temperature.

Your appestat must monitor many different chemical processes to keep you eating healthy amounts. It probably keeps track of a substance called *glucose*, or blood sugar. When your glucose level is low, you feel hungry. When it's high, you feel satisfied. Your brain may also sense tiny changes in body temperature after you eat, and start the signal that says "I've had enough." Scientists would like to know more about how the appetite is regulated. This knowledge could help them treat conditions such as obesity, which makes people dangerously fat, and other eating problems.

Your imagination plays a role in stimulating your appestat, too. Close your eyes and picture your favorite food in your mind. Is your stomach growling yet?

Why do I burp and get the hiccups?

Have you ever given a baby a bottle? It's an important job, and it needs to be done right. Erin learned the art of feeding an infant when she got a summer job baby-sitting for a six-month-old boy. Erin soon found out that when babies drink their bottles, they like

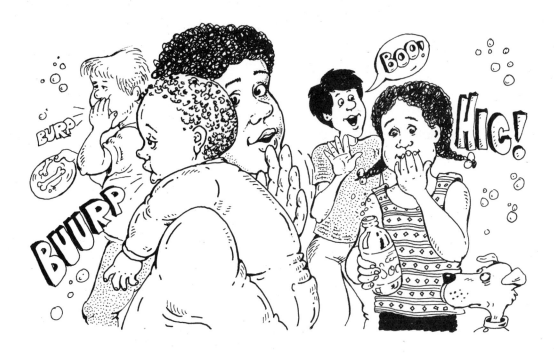

to be cuddled. She also found out that it's important to make sure the baby burps after he drinks.

"Just pat his back gently," the baby's mom explained. Erin tried it, holding the little boy on her shoulder as she stroked his back.

"Urp!" he said. Both Erin and the baby's mom laughed.

"That was a good one," the baby's mom said.

Erin thought it was pretty funny that the baby was being praised for burping. When Erin burps, her mom says, "Say excuse me, Erin, please."

A burp isn't really all that rude, although the sound does offend some people. It's just your body's way of getting rid of swallowed air. If you gobble a container of French fries, you swallow air along with the food. Before long, you may feel like a burp is on its way.

You have two separate pipes in your throat. Your *windpipe* carries air into your lungs when you breathe. Your *esophagus* takes food to your stomach. When you're eating, the opening to your windpipe closes automatically to keep food or drink from going down, but your esophagus stays open, of course. Otherwise your food wouldn't be able to get to your stomach. As the food goes

51

down, air goes down, too. The extra air in your stomach can give you an unpleasant sense of fullness, but burping relieves that feeling.

When you drink carbonated soft drinks, you swallow lots of the gas bubbles that give the drink its fizz. Those bubbles can also lead to burps. Some foods that have a lot of air mixed into them to make them light—such as whipped cream—can also make you burp. Talking a lot as you eat can lead to swallowing extra air, and to extra burping. Many adults think that burping is rude, so you might try to keep the gobbling, talking with your mouth full, and soda guzzling under control.

Babies need to be burped because they swallow a lot of air with the liquid they suck in. If the air travels down into the stomach, instead of popping back out the mouth, it can cause the baby pain. This happens because the air expands, or grows larger, as it warms up inside the baby's stomach. It pushes the walls of the stomach outward—and that hurts! There's even a medical name for this condition; it's called *aerophagia*. "Aero" means air. "Phagia" means eating. The name shows that the baby got its stomachache from eating air.

If you have ever been around a baby with a stomachache, you know they can yell their heads off. Helping a baby get rid of the extra air by patting it lightly on the back can go a long way toward preventing that problem. No wonder mothers praise babies who burp.

Babies, like kids and adults, sometimes get the hiccups, too. Like burps, the noises can happen at embarrassing moments. Hiccuping happens when your normal breathing pattern gets interrupted. Experts aren't sure why this happens. The diaphragm—a powerful muscle that helps you breathe—gets out of rhythm with the rest of your breathing muscles. It sends an unusual gust of air rushing into the lungs. At the same time, your brain tells your tongue and the upper part of your throat to clamp down to stop the rush of air. As the diaphragm pushes and the tongue clamps, the air jets across your vocal cords, and you make that weird sound we call a hiccup. There are many, many different "cures" that people try—holding their breath, drinking water out of the rim of a glass, putting a paper bag over their heads—but the best cure for the *hic-hic-hic-hic* sound appears to be time. You just have to wait for them to go away! And they do.

Why do I have an appendix?

Grace, a ten-year-old, was getting ready to go off on vacation when she developed a bad stomachache. It felt different from other stomachaches she'd had before.

Grace's stomachache started as pain in the area of her belly button. Later it moved down to her lower right side, above the hip bone. It really hurt, especially when she moved or coughed. Gracie told her parents about the pain, and they took her to the doctor right away.

Gracie's doctor checked her symptoms. She felt sick to her stomach. She had also developed a high fever. The doctor decided Gracie had *appendicitis*.

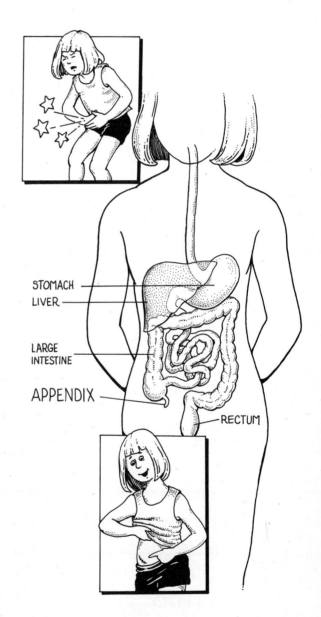

STOMACH
LIVER
LARGE INTESTINE
APPENDIX
RECTUM

When they heard the news, Gracie's parents decided to postpone the family's vacation. Gracie was admitted to the hospital for an *appendectomy*. After her operation, when she was feeling completely well again, they set off for the beach at last. Gracie felt like she'd really earned her vacation.

When you get a bad stomachache, do you ever wonder if you have appendicitis? Many people, both grown-ups and kids, do worry about it—and for good reason. Appendicitis can be a pretty serious illness unless it is treated quickly.

What is an appendix, anyway? Its name gives you a clue. The medical name for this body part is the *vermiform appendix*, or "worm-shaped attachment." Appendix means "added on" or "attached to." That's a pretty accurate description. Your appendix is a little dead-end tube or sac about three inches long that dangles from the lowest part of your large intestine. It's ordinarily located on the lower right side, though in some people it's on the other side.

The appendix doesn't seem to have an important job to do in the human body. But while people apparently don't need their appendixes, some animals do. In rabbits, cows, and some other plant-eating animals, the appendix helps break down the tough fibers in the leaves and grass they eat. Some experts think that a long time ago, primitive human beings might have had much larger appendixes than we do today, because they ate more tough plant material.

In humans today, the main thing the appendix does is sometimes cause trouble. Sometimes a small, hard particle of undigested food on its way through your intestines may drop into the hollow inside of your appendix.

If the particle gets stuck, it may block up the entrance to the appendix. Bacteria that normally live in your intestine get trapped inside the appendix. Under normal conditions, bacteria help break down the food you eat. But when they're trapped inside the appendix, they start to cause trouble. They continue doing what bacteria do best: multiplying. The number of bacteria inside the appendix gets larger and larger. This irritates the appendix, making it swell up and turn hot and red. This is the medical problem called appendicitis.

If the condition gets serious, surgery is needed. A doctor has to remove the appendix before it bursts. If the appendix bursts inside the patient, a very serious infection will spread into the body.

An English doctor performed the first appendectomy in 1736—more than two centuries ago. Today doctors are still doing a similar operation, although they use much more modern methods. Each year in the United States between 200,000 and 300,000 people have their appendixes removed. Most of the people who have their appendixes out are between the ages of five and thirty, but the condition is more common in people over age fifteen.

How do my kidneys work?

Have you ever built something? Let's say you take shop at school, and your project is to construct a wooden birdhouse. You start with raw materials—wood, nails, glue, and paint—and you go to work.

As you build, you saw off scraps of wood and make sawdust. You bend a couple of nails and throw them aside. You use an old rag to wipe off a little extra paint. When your project is finished, you pick up all the bits of leftover material and toss them away. Those scraps of lumber and dirty rags are the waste produced as you use energy and materials to build a birdhouse.

Almost any job—whether it's making scrambled eggs, building a barn, or doing your homework—creates waste products. When

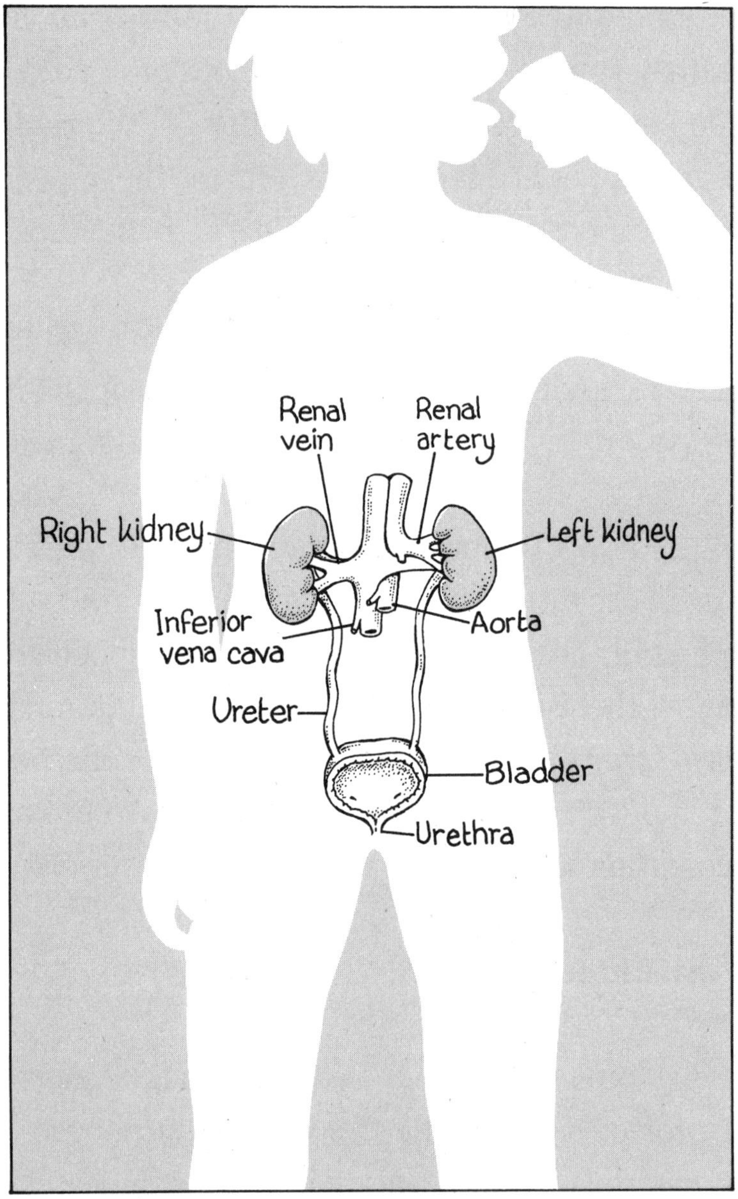
Renal vein
Renal artery
Right kidney
Left kidney
Inferior vena cava
Aorta
Ureter
Bladder
Urethra

the task is done, you have to get rid of the eggshells, the leftover lumber, or the balled-up pieces of scratch paper.

The job of keeping the human body going creates waste products, too. These products are chemicals your cells give off as they burn energy. To stay healthy, you have to get rid of the chemicals, which can be harmful in large amounts. That's where your kidneys come in.

If you reach around and touch the lowest ribs on your back, your hands will be about where your kidneys are. You have two of them, one on each side of your body. They're located deep inside you, protected by a cushion of fat cells and the armor of your rib cage. They're not very big—each is about the size of a human fist and weighs about a quarter of a pound—but they do an enormous job. They keep you from poisoning yourself with the waste products your own cells create.

You might think of the kidneys as a pair of nonstop washing machines for your blood. Each minute, about a quart of blood passes through the kidneys and comes out clean. In a lifetime, your kidneys wash your blood over and over again—more than 1 million gallons' worth. That's enough to fill a small lake.

Your kidneys may not be very fancy-looking or very large, but they have an amazing amount of equipment packed inside them. In fact, these vital organs are one of the most complex parts of your body. Your brain is a more complicated structure—but the kidneys come in second.

Each kidney contains a network of tiny tubes and bundles of blood vessels that act as filters for your blood. These tiny tubes are called *nephrons*. Each kidney contains about 1 million nephrons.

The kidneys' blood-washing business is important. Each day, your kidneys constantly filter your blood. Poisonous substances that would make you very sick or even kill you are washed out of the body and carried away from the kidneys in a watery fluid called *urine*. The urine collects in a bag called the *bladder*. When the bladder gets full, it stretches. This action alerts nerve cells, which relay a message to your brain. It says, "Time to go to the bathroom," where you get rid of the urine and flush it away. Every day, the human body processes between one and two quarts of urine.

Your kidneys are more than just a human washing machine.

They also help keep the chemical balance in your body correct. Regulating the body's chemistry is a very complicated job.

Having two kidneys gives people a kind of built-in insurance policy. In healthy people, each kidney is at work all the time. But sometimes an illness or an injury can harm one kidney. Luckily, the other one can continue to work hard enough to keep the person well.

If both kidneys are damaged, medical technology can help. For about thirty years now, doctors have been able to transplant kidneys from one person to another. Or a piece of equipment called a *kidney dialysis machine* can be used to wash a patient's blood when the kidneys have stopped doing their job.

You probably don't give your kidneys much thought. Luckily, you don't have to. They work automatically. Even as you sleep, your own personal cleanup crew is on the job.

Why do I get thirsty?

On a warm day you run in from the playground and head for the water fountain yelling, "I'm thirsty!" At home, you munch on a salty snack, say, "I'm thirsty," and open the refrigerator. In bed, you wake up in the middle of the night, mumble, "I'm thirsty," hoping your mom or dad will stumble in with a drink of water for you.

Then there are other times when you think you can't possibly drink another drop. After you have gulped half a bottle of juice, or drunk a tall glass of water to wash down a pill, you may not like the idea of pouring more liquid into your body.

Thirst—or the lack of thirst—is your body's way of making sure your cells contain exactly the right amount of water to work well.

The part of your body you can't see is called your *internal environment*. It's pretty damp. In fact, it's more than half water. To be healthy, your internal environment has to be just right—not

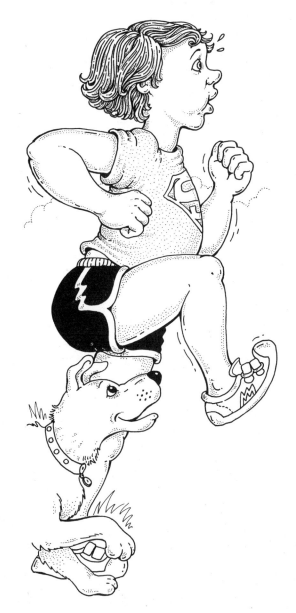

too wet, not too dry. So your body comes equipped with a system that keeps track of the amount of water inside.

When you think about the water inside your body, you may think that you're like a bottle half filled with liquid. It's not really like that at all. Much of your weight comes from water, but it's not sloshing around like some kind of puddle. It's spread throughout the billions of cells that form your body. Some of the water is inside your cells. The rest of it bathes the outside of the cells, creating a healthy environment for them.

The amount of water in your cells changes all the time. As you breathe, you send some water vapor out of your body. When you sweat, you get rid of more water. Over the course of the day, you lose nearly two quarts of water when you go to the bathroom. All that lost water has to be replaced—so you drink.

The feeling of thirst is your body's way of letting you know when it's time to drink something. Inside you, your nerves and brain work together to monitor the amount of water in your cells. When the level gets low, you experience that dry feeling in the back of your throat that makes you want something to drink.

One way your nerves and brain keep track of the water in your cells is by measuring the amount of salt mixed with it. All human beings must have some salt inside them to stay alive. The salt and water mixture in your cells must stay at a certain level to keep your body working. If the balance of salt and other chemicals in your internal water supply is not right, you may get sick.

One of the things salt does is to help your blood keep circulating. When the level of water in your body drops, the salt level goes up. Nerve cells sense this and sound the "time-for-a-drink" alarm. The water you drink mixes in with the salt to make a weaker—and healthier—bath for the cells. That's why eating salty foods makes you thirsty. Your body has to drink more water to dilute the salt.

When your brain senses that there's too much water around your cells, they start a different process. This one involves producing hormones, which are the chemical messengers that speed to the kidneys. Your kidneys are then alerted to make more urine, which washes excess water out when you go to the bathroom.

Without water, you would last only a few days. So drink up. Like the oxygen in the air you breathe, water is essential for life. Water bathes your cells, carries nutrients to the places in the body that need them, and keeps your body temperature at a healthy level.

3

SENSATIONAL SENSES

As you go through your day, your five senses let you know what's going on around you. This chapter answers some questions about how the senses of touch, hearing, sight, smell, and taste work, and why they're so important to survival.

What's so funny about tickling?

When you tickle a baby's tummy, you're usually rewarded with a grin and a giggle. If you're ticklish yourself, you may get teased by your friends sometimes.

If someone walks up to you wiggling his fingers, you may start laughing before he even touches you. Then when you're actually being tickled, you scream with laughter and fall down on the floor. "Boy, are you sensitive," your friend might say.

Your friend is right. You are sensitive—and it's your sense of touch that's at work as you wriggle and laugh when being tickled.

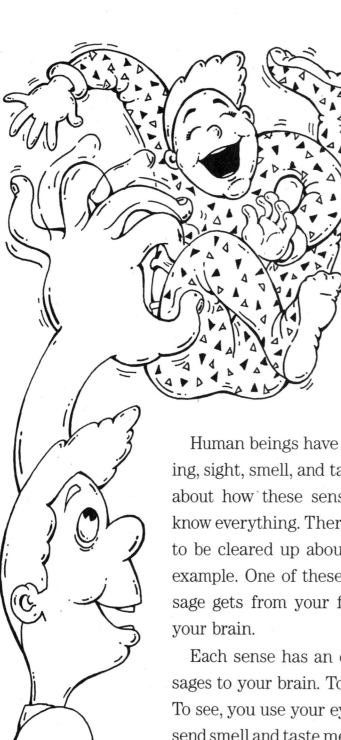

Human beings have five senses—touch, hearing, sight, smell, and taste. Scientists know a lot about how these senses work, but they don't know everything. There are still some mysteries to be cleared up about the sense of touch, for example. One of these is how the "tickle" message gets from your friend's wiggly fingers to your brain.

Each sense has an organ it uses to get messages to your brain. To hear, you use your ears. To see, you use your eyes. Your nose and mouth send smell and taste messages to your brain. And you sense touch with your skin.

In your skin, there are small bundles of cells called *receptors*. They're called receptors because they receive messages. Your body contains an enormous network of different kinds of receptors. Some of them can sense temperature. Others sense pressure. Others sense pain.

Let's say you've just awakened in the morning. Your head is cradled by a feather pillow. As you turn over, one of the feathers pops out of a hole in the seam and lands on your face. A receptor in your skin sends a signal to your brain about the feather. The message? "Soft."

Next, your mother calls to you to get moving or you'll be late for school. You peer out the window and see the gray winter day outside. You pull the blankets back over your shoulders and snuggle down. All over your skin, receptors pick up a message. It says: "warm."

But you have to go to school, so you climb out of bed, and put your bare feet on the floor. Two more messages flash to your brain. They say: "cold" and "hard." Then as you shuffle off to the bathroom you get a splinter in your foot. The message this time? "Ouch! Pain."

At the breakfast table your sister leans over and tickles you under the arm. "Smile," she says. You can't help it. You're ticklish, and you laugh.

The receptor that sent that "tickle" message to your brain is a special kind. The nerve endings that sense tickles and itches are called *free nerve endings*. You have lots of free nerve endings in your body, and researchers are still at work trying to figure out exactly what role they play in your sense of touch.

Some touch receptors are extremely sensitive. They can feel the movement of the fine hairs on your forearm, for example. They can sense a touch so brief that it lasts only a tenth of a second. They can also feel longer, stronger touches such as a big bear hug. Sensitive pain receptors send signals to your brain so fast that you pull your hand away from a hot stove even before you know you've touched it.

Scientists used to think that the tickle reaction was caused by mild activity around the pain receptors. But now they think that ticklish feelings come from nerve endings in the very outer layers of your skin. When these nerve endings are bothered, they cause that familiar wriggling and giggling reaction—in some people. Other people aren't ticklish at all.

How do my ears work?

Bang! A car door slams shut. A taxi driver blasts a warning on a horn. In the middle of the street, a construction worker *rat-a-tat-tats* at the pavement with a jackhammer. People shout to each other over the noise of the traffic.

These are the sounds you might hear at a busy city intersection. In the country, you would hear different sounds. You could listen to leaves rustling in the breeze or bees buzzing in flowers. You might hear a dog barking way off on the other side of a wide field.

Sound—whether it's loud or soft—travels through the air in waves. You can hear because your ears are built to pick up the sound waves. The waves enter your ear, where they are translated into nerve signals that your brain understands.

Look at a friend's ear. The first thing you will see is the *outer ear.* It gathers sound waves and passes them into the *inner ear.* When you look at your friend's ear, you can see a dark hole leading into the head. That's the *ear canal.* It leads to the important working parts of the ear, which you can't see.

A small piece of skin stretches across the opening between the ear canal and the inner ear. This is the *eardrum,* and it has a very important job. When sound waves from the outside strike the eardrum, it starts vibrating. The vibrations pass into a tiny bone on the other side of the eardrum. This bone, called the *hammer,* attaches to two other tiny bones, the *anvil* and the *stirrup.* The

64

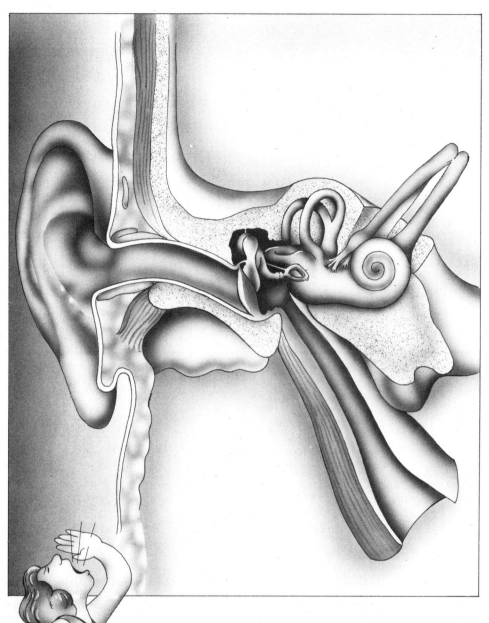

stirrup is the smallest bone in your body—no larger than a grain of rice.

Let's say you whisper something to your friend. The three connected bones pass sound waves from her eardrum to her inner ear. There, a snail-shaped part of the inner ear takes over the job of changing sound waves into nerve signals. This part, called the *cochlea*, is carved right into the bone that forms the skull. There is liquid inside the cochlea, which picks up the vibrations passed from the eardrum. The liquid quivers and stimulates thousands of tiny nerve cells that line the cochlea. The cells send messages to the part of your brain that's in charge of hearing, and your friend hears your whisper.

Your ears are very sensitive, so they are equipped with special things designed for protection. The wax that lines your ear canal keeps dirt from getting in. The wax in your ears is necessary for good health. You shouldn't ever try to scrape it out with a cotton swab or any other object. You could damage your delicate eardrum.

The bone that surrounds your hardworking inner ear is the hardest bone in your body. It's a kind of armor to protect the ear.

Passages called *eustachian tubes* connect your ears and your throat. The tubes open and close at different times to keep the pressure inside your ears normal. When you go up or down in an airplane and your ears "pop," it's a sign that these tubes are doing their job.

But as most kids know, ears can be troublesome. Doctors report that half of all children have earaches at one time or another. Most earaches are caused by infections inside the ear. The infection may come from germs that travel up the eustachian tubes when you have a cold or sore throat. The infection may make your inner ear swollen and painful.

Very loud noises, such as explosions, can cause hearing loss. So can listening to very loud music for a long time. So turn that stereo down a little. Your ears need to last a lifetime.

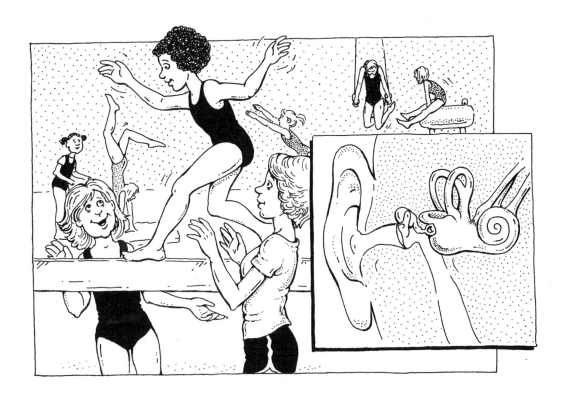

When I tried to walk on the balance beam in gym class, I fell off. How do people keep their balance?

Gymnastics is a lot of fun, but some of the routines are hard—especially walking on the balance beam.

Cheryl is learning gymnastics with her fifth-grade class. The first time she tried the balance beam, she was really nervous. Her teacher and a classmate acted as her "spotters." They stood on either side to help Cheryl if she lost her balance.

Once she got up on the beam, Cheryl discovered that she could walk on it pretty well—so long as she went slowly. About halfway across she lost her balance and had to jump off. She got right back up, and although she wobbled more than she walked she made it all the way to the end. "You've got a good sense of balance," her gym teacher said.

Most of the time, you keep your balance without even thinking about it. But it wasn't always that easy. Take a look at a toddler who has just learned how to walk. You'll notice that he staggers around, has a hard time walking in a straight line, and falls down a lot. Developing balance and coordination for walking upright takes practice.

Where is your sense of balance, anyway? It's located in a place you might not expect—your inner ear. Your balance-control equipment is found right next to the cochlea, the liquid-filled part of your ear that passes sound to the eardrum. Two little liquid-filled bags called the *utricle* and the *saccule* keep track of your sense of up and down. Next to the utricle and saccule there are three loops called the *semicircular canals*. They're filled with liquid, too. The semicircular canals are in charge of your sense of direction—that is, whether you're moving forward, backward, or from side to side.

This whole system for keeping you balanced is called the *vestibular apparatus*. Each part of the system contains bundles of nerves. As you move, the fluid in the inner ear swirls or tips, depending on what you're doing. The motion of the liquid affects the nerves, and they send signals on to your brain.

Your brain's role in keeping you balanced is complicated. It uses the information from your inner ear to position the parts of your body so that you don't fall over. When Cheryl walked along the beam, she found it easier to stay upright if she moved her arms up and down by her sides. Her brain told her that using her arms that way would keep her upright. And it worked!

Most of the time, your sense of balance does its job perfectly. But when you do something unusual—such as spin around on your ice skates or stand on your head—the sensitive system gets upset. The liquid in the inner ear sloshes around, and your brain gets confusing signals. If your sense of balance could talk, it might ask, "Am I up or down? Am I going forward or backward? Which way is up?"

When your sense of balance is thrown off, you feel dizzy. As the sloshing in your inner ear calms down, that unsettling feeling goes away. Sometimes just a little dizziness can be pleasant. That's why kids like to go up and down on playground swings. But if you have ever swung too long, you know that dizziness can make you feel queasy, too.

Have you ever noticed that when you spin around, you still feel the movement even after you stop? That's because the liquid in your inner ear keeps swirling for a few moments after your body stops moving. It keeps sending the message "you're spinning" to your brain. But when the liquid slows down and gets level again, your sense of balance catches up with your body, and you feel normal.

When Cheryl was up on that balance beam, she was asking her body to perform an unusual task. We don't normally walk on such a narrow path. The strange situation caused some disturbance in her inner ear. When she lost her balance, the fluids had sloshed around so much that her body couldn't keep up with the "stay upright" signals. When she got back on and made it to the end of the beam, her sense of balance was doing a better job at keeping her body in position. The fluids in her inner ear didn't slosh, and she made it to the end of the beam successfully.

Why do some people throw up when they go on long car trips?

Many people suffer from car sickness, or from other kinds of motion sickness such as airsickness or seasickness. For those people, travel isn't much fun. Being in an interesting new place is great, but getting there is terrible. Some people even avoid traveling because of motion sickness.

Some people don't get motion sickness at all. Some unlucky

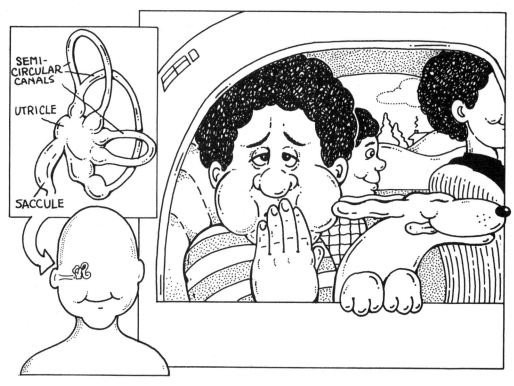

people get it even on very short trips, such as a ride on an escalator. People with bad motion sickness may even throw up.

To understand motion sickness, you have to start with a part of your body hidden deep inside your head. Like dizziness, motion sickness is caused by disturbances in the inner ear.

Wait a minute—inside your head? You'd think that a sickness that made you feel queasy would start in your stomach.

Motion sickness sometimes does end up making you sick to your stomach. But it begins in your balancing equipment—the utricle, saccule, and semicircular canals in your inner ear—where feelings of dizziness also begin.

But what does all this have to do with feeling queasy when you're sitting in the backseat of a car on the way to your grandmother's house?

A lot. Even though you're not spinning around as you travel along the highway—unless your parents have a very weird car—you are in constant motion. Objects outside the car move by, and your eyes dart from side to side, keeping the trees or cows or road signs in focus as you go. Your brain has a lot to do: It must constantly process the signals from your eyes and sort out whether you're sitting still or moving—when you're actually doing both.

During the trip, your brain gets mixed signals, and continues to get them so long as the car is in motion. Once the signals get confused, you may experience a similar feeling to the one you get when you spin around. The medical name for this feeling is *vertigo*. You call it dizziness. But whatever it's called, it makes you feel awful.

The fast cure for motion sickness is pretty easy to figure out. Just stop moving. If you're on a pitching boat, you'll feel better after you go ashore. If you're airsick, you'll be cured by coming in for a landing.

But you can't avoid taking trips, and you wouldn't want to. Doctors have found that some medicines work well to treat the symptoms of motion sickness. Like many medications, however, drugs that fight motion sickness may not be good for children. Or they may have side effects that are just as unpleasant as the motion sickness. But for some people who get very bad motion sickness, medicine is the only solution. Your pediatrician should decide if you need to use medicine.

If your motion sickness isn't too bad, try keeping a window open—if you're in a car—and listening to the radio to distract yourself. If you feel sick, try lying down and keeping your head still. It may help to suck on an ice cube or drink some cola or eat some crackers. Don't try to read or look at the passing scenery. This will just make the poor inner ear and brain more confused.

In a car, ask the driver to make frequent stops to let your inner ear get back to doing its usual great balancing act. It may not be much comfort when you're feeling queasy now, but many kids get over their car sickness as they get older.

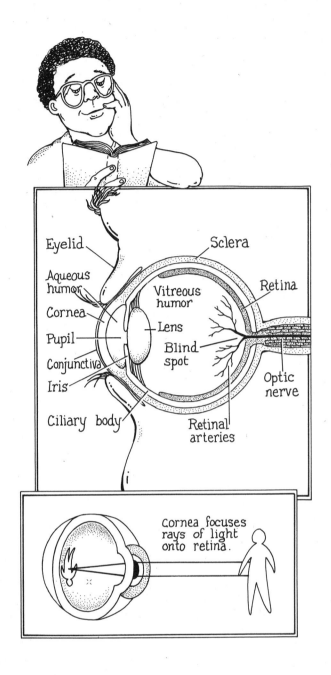

Cornea focuses
rays of light
onto retina.

How do I see?

Each morning when you wake up and open your eyes, a pair of the most remarkable parts of your body go to work. When you are awake your eyes constantly gather information and send it on to your brain. Take a break from reading this page and look around the room where you are sitting. Your eyes not only show you all the objects in the room, they also show you how much light is in the room, what color everything is, and how close or far away things are.

The process of seeing takes place in a fraction of a second, and it happens automatically. You don't have to decide to see—if your eyes are open, you just do it. But a lot of things happen during that split second that it takes to look around.

Your eyes come equipped with several different parts. Your eyes are shaped like Ping-Pong balls and are about the same size. They're well protected by your bony skull, and by your eyelids and eyelashes.

A tough coating called the *sclera* covers each eyeball. This is the part of your eye that looks white. A little hole in the sclera lets in light. You can see this hole, called the *pupil,* as a black circle in the middle of the colored part of your eye.

The colored part of your eye, called the *iris,* contains special muscles to open and shut the pupil. You have probably noticed that your pupils are sometimes tiny dots, and sometimes larger black circles. In very bright light, the pupil of the eye closes down, the way you might pull a blind down on a window. In dimmer light, the pupil opens wide to allow more light into the eye. You can see the pupil in action if you go to a movie one afternoon with your friends. Their pupils will be wide open in the dim light of the movie theater. But back outside, their pupils will shut down to pinpoints in the bright light of afternoon. Your pupils will do exactly the same thing.

A see-through disk called the *cornea* covers the outside of your pupil and iris. It collects light and sends it through the pupil to the inside of your eyeball. That's where seeing starts.

Once light rays pass through your pupil, they are focused by your *lens*. This part of your eye looks a lot like the lens of a magnifying glass, but it's smaller and very flexible. It can change shape to focus the light rays coming in from outside. After focusing, the lens projects the light onto the sensitive surface at the back of the eyeball.

The light-sensitive surface is called the *retina*. An amazing thing happens on the retina. The light rays from outside form an upside-down image, or picture, on the back of the eye. Then special cells change the picture into nerve signals, which rush off to your brain. The brain turns the picture right-side up, and you see.

All of this equipment sounds pretty complicated—and it is. Your eyes are very sensitive and complex. Sometimes they don't work exactly right. But for most people who need help in seeing, glasses or contact lenses can be prescribed. The lenses or glasses are designed to help your eyes focus images clearly.

My friend has a green shirt but he says it's gray. Why can't he see green?

Green is a common color. But some people can't see it because they are color-blind. They see normally, but their eyes don't recognize certain colors. They may be able to see blue, but not red or green. Instead, things that are red or green appear in shades of gray.

To understand color blindness, you need to know how the eye works. Light comes into the eye through the small, dark hole in the center called the pupil. The light passes through a lens. The lens focuses the light, and projects it onto the back of the eyeball. This part of the eye, called the retina, contains special cells that are sensitive to light.

When you look at something, the cells in your retina respond by sending chemical signals to the brain. The signals travel along the *optic nerve* to the *visual cortex*—the part of your brain that is in

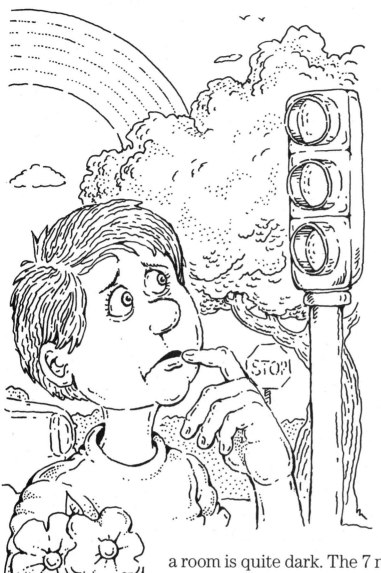

charge of vision. There the nerve signals are translated into an image—and you see.

Millions of nerve cells are located in the retina. Some of the nerves are called *rods;* others are called *cones.* The 100 million rods in each eye are sensitive in dim light and allow you to see shades of gray. They make the adjustments that make it possible for you to see what is around you even when a room is quite dark. The 7 million cone cells in each eye are sensitive to different colors. They can only see color in bright light, though. That's why colorful things look gray or black when you look at them in dim light.

The cone cells in your eyes come in three different types. Each type responds to a different color—to red, green, or blue. Your brain combines those three basic colors into a rainbow of different shades.

Sometimes one color is strongest in the object you're looking at. When you look at a stop sign, for example, your red cones react strongly to the color, and you recognize it as red. Color-blind people who don't see red also recognize stop signs, of course—but by their shape, not their color.

People who are color-blind are missing certain types of cone cells. They may see blue and green, but not red. If all three types of cone cells are missing, the person sees only black, white, and shades of gray. But total color blindness is rare. Confusing red with green is much more common.

Everyone is color-blind at the beginning of life. That's because cone cells don't develop in the eyes until a baby is about six to eight months old. At that age, babies begin to get interested in looking at colorful toys and pictures.

Color blindness is more common in men. In the United States, about eight of every one hundred men are color-blind. About one in every two hundred women is color-blind. Color blindness is something people inherit from their parents. Like hair color or eye color, it is a genetic trait. If one or both parents is color-blind, then the chances of having a color-blind child go up.

People who are color-blind may not even know it. A color-blind person may have a green shirt and think it's gray, or a red shirt and think it's green. But being color-blind doesn't cause too much trouble.

Eye doctors use special vision tests to discover if people are color-blind. The tests contain letters, numbers, or images made up of lots of dots. The dots forming the number or letter might be green, surrounded by a pattern of red dots. In that case, a person who can't see green won't be able to read the test. All that would be visible would be a bunch of red dots.

There's nothing to be done about being color-blind. Luckily, it's not an uncomfortable condition. It's not particularly dangerous, either. People who are color-blind have to learn other ways to recognize things such as traffic lights and other color-coded sig-

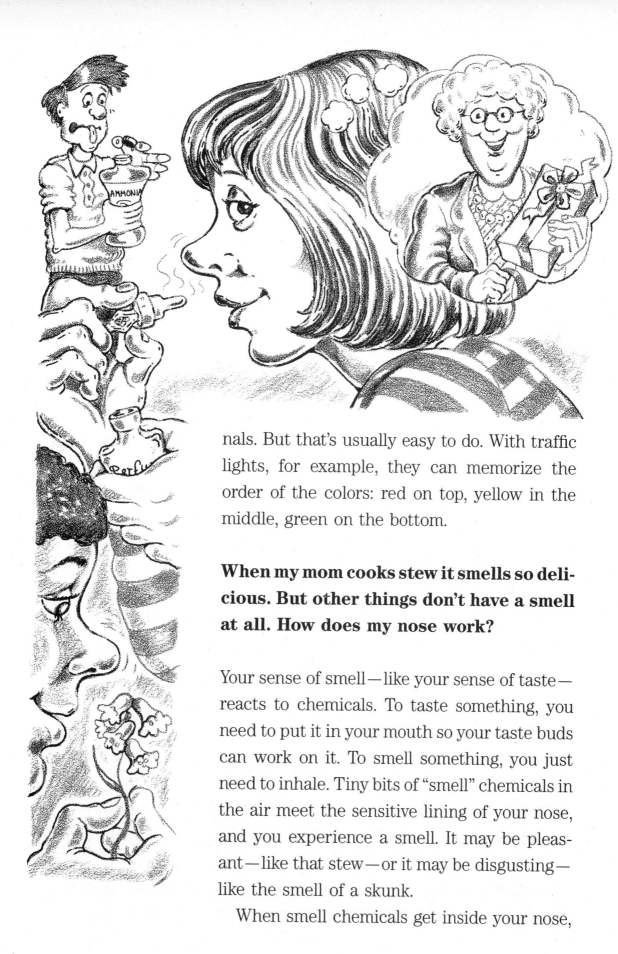

nals. But that's usually easy to do. With traffic lights, for example, they can memorize the order of the colors: red on top, yellow in the middle, green on the bottom.

When my mom cooks stew it smells so delicious. But other things don't have a smell at all. How does my nose work?

Your sense of smell—like your sense of taste—reacts to chemicals. To taste something, you need to put it in your mouth so your taste buds can work on it. To smell something, you just need to inhale. Tiny bits of "smell" chemicals in the air meet the sensitive lining of your nose, and you experience a smell. It may be pleasant—like that stew—or it may be disgusting—like the smell of a skunk.

When smell chemicals get inside your nose,

they dissolve in the damp mucus inside. Then the smell chemicals stimulate small patches of nerve endings in the upper part of each nostril. The patches are small, but they're packed with nerve endings. Each nostril has 10 million of them! If you like a smell, you may sniff several times over. That puts more of the smell chemicals in touch with your nerve endings.

Scientists think that we can identify about ten thousand different odors. This sense can be a lifesaver—smelling smoke, for example, can warn you to get out of the house fast and call the fire department. It can tell you that the milk you were planning to drink is sour. Your sense of smell can also get you prepared for a meal. The good smell of the stew in your kitchen starts your mouth watering, and you'll soon be using that saliva to help digest your food.

The sense of smell is still pretty mysterious; scientists just aren't certain how it works. They do know that some smells call up vivid memories. You've probably had that experience yourself. For instance, the smell of pine trees may remind you of your camp in Maine. The smell of a particular perfume may remind you of your grandmother. The smell of white glue may make you think back to your kindergarten days. Scientists think this link between smell and memory happens because your "smell" nerve endings connect with the part of your brain that stores memory.

You may think you have a sensitive nose. But your smell cells cover patches less than 1 square inch. A dog may have 10 square inches of smell cells in its nose!

My dad says I have a "sweet tooth." Why do I like sweet things so much?

Having a "sweet tooth" is a slang expression for loving sugary things. But it's not your teeth that notice the sweet taste of a gooey

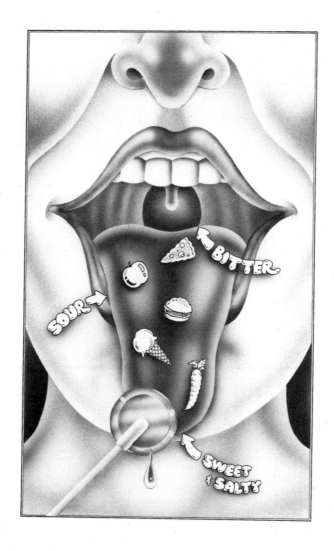

candy bar. In fact, your teeth would be better off without the sugar in the candy. You taste the sweetness through *taste buds* on your tongue.

Under a microscope, taste buds look a bit like flower buds. If you look at your tongue in the mirror, you'll notice that it isn't smooth. The tiny bumps that cover it are your taste buds. They pick up chemical signals from the food you eat. These signals say "sweet," "sour," "salty," and "bitter." Those are the four taste groups that your tongue can experience. Many foods combine these different tastes—and add a pleasant smell to make an even more appealing flavor.

The way a food smells is an important part of the experience you have when you eat it. You can find this out by doing a few simple taste tests in your kitchen. Check page 129 to find out how to do the experiment.

You taste different flavors with different parts of your tongue. With the tip, you taste sweet and salty things. You taste sour things most strongly with the outer edges of the tongue. You taste bitter things on the back of the tongue.

Scientists have wondered why people enjoy sweet-tasting things so much. Experiments have shown that babies suck longest and hardest on bottles of sweet liquid. That's a good thing, since the milk they drink from their mothers' bodies when they're nursing is sweet.

Another possible explanation for a "sweet tooth" has to do with the days long ago when people lived on the food they gathered. Healthful fruits, nuts, and berries often have a sweet taste. But berries and plants that contain poison taste bitter. So the taste buds' ability to detect bitterness may have served as a warning system. If something tasted good, it was probably safe to eat. If it tasted bitter, it was a good idea to spit it out.

Dr. Diana Spillman, a scientist who studies taste at Florida State University, has found that young children have more taste buds than adults do. Before age five, children have taste buds on the lips and the inside of the mouth as well as on the tongue. As kids grow, the number of taste buds on the tongue slowly decreases. As an adult, you'll have between nine and ten thousand taste buds left—which is still plenty. Dr. Spillman thinks the extra taste buds kids have may explain why they like sweets so much.

Even so, it's a good idea to develop the taste for other foods, too. Our bodies need some sugar. But too much of it can cause tooth decay and other health problems. So the next time you reach for a candy bar, remember that your taste buds might like to experience a carrot or a peanut butter sandwich just as much.

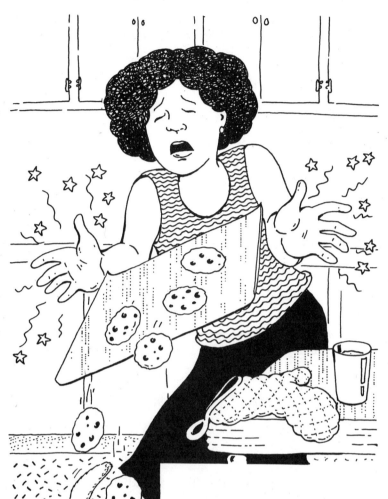

Why does it hurt to get a burn or a cut?

OW! You try to pick up a cookie sheet from the kitchen counter, and it's still hot. You drop the pan, and the cookies fall to the floor. You stick your hand in your mouth to cool it off, and heave a sigh of relief that you weren't badly burned.

During the few moments that it took for you to realize that you'd grabbed a hot pan, your body was busy. It was using pain as an alarm system to tell you to let go of the pan before you hurt yourself badly.

When you touched the pan, your body didn't

stop to consider that you'd ruin a fresh batch of cookies by dropping them. Your body's first concern was protecting itself. In fact, the physical reflex, or automatic reaction, that made you drop the pan happened before your body even had time to send a pain signal to your brain.

As soon as the nerves in your fingers felt the heat in the metal cookie sheet, a message flashed to your brain, ordering you to drop the pan as fast as possible. Other nerve signals told the brain, "This hurts!"

Nerve endings in your skin sense touch, pressure, and pain. Your nerves allow you to feel things, from the soft, pleasant touch of your parents' hands, to the short, sharp pain of a needle when you get a shot.

We all know that pain is unpleasant. But it can be useful, too. In addition to serving as a warning signal in this cookie-sheet crisis, the pain may help protect you in the future. The next time you see a pan of cookies on the counter, you'll probably think twice about picking it up without using an oven mitt.

Pain acts as a warning system in many different situations. If you break a bone, pain tells you that the injury is serious and needs attention right away. The pain, headache, and fever of a bad cold or the flu tell you that you should lie down and rest, allowing your body time to heal. The pain of a stomachache tells you it's time to stop eating those apples off your neighbor's tree.

Sometimes you feel pain when something goes wrong inside your body. You can't see the problem the way you can see a cut or a bruise, but you can feel it. This pain warning system tells you about illnesses such as appendicitis.

Pain forces you to react. When you feel pain, you don't just go on with life as usual. You go to your father or mother or the school nurse and say, "It hurts. Please do something to make it feel better."

4

GETTING SICK, STAYING WELL

Most of the time, human beings are healthy and strong. But sometimes things go wrong, and people catch illnesses. This chapter answers some questions about why people get sick, and how their bodies fight to get better again.

Why do I go to a pediatrician instead of a plain old doctor for my checkups?

Pediatricians are special doctors just for kids. They have received special training to make them experts at taking care of children. Another kind of doctor—a family practitioner—is also trained to care for children.

Right after you were born you had your first checkup by a pediatrician, although you don't remember it. The specialist who helped your mother as you were born handed you over to the pediatrician to make sure you were healthy.

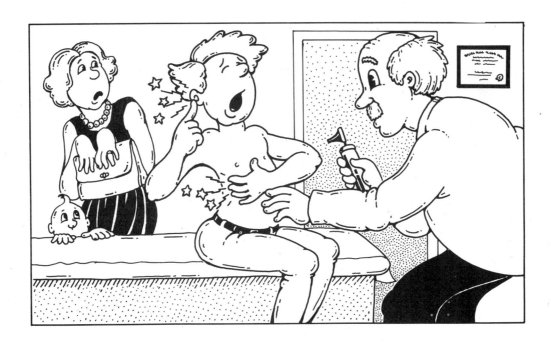

At your first checkup, your pediatrician may have decided you were in great shape, and sent you right off to the nursery or to your mother's room to begin two important infant activities: eating and sleeping.

But if you showed any signs of needing extra care—and about 15 percent of newborns do—your doctor may have decided you needed to spend some time in an enclosed bed called an *incubator*. The air inside an incubator can be kept at a constant temperature to keep the baby warm. When babies are in incubators, nurses and doctors keep track of their heart rate and their breathing.

After you were born, your mom's doctor decided when she was well enough to go home. Your pediatrician made the same decision about you. Once you were home, your parents kept a close eye on your growth and development. They took you to the pediatrician on a regular schedule. The doctor kept track of your height and weight, gave you shots to protect you from common childhood illnesses such as measles, and generally kept track of how you were doing.

Pediatricians keep looking after the growth and development of children through the early years of their lives. Even teenagers go to pediatricians, although many doctors keep separate waiting rooms for their older patients. You may continue to see the same pediatrician until you go away to college. Some doctors like to keep track of their patients until they're twenty-one.

Dr. Francis M. Palumbo is the director of the children's center at Georgetown University Hospital in Washington, D.C. He thinks pediatricians are special people. Palumbo believes that many doctors decide to specialize in pediatrics because they like kids. "We're trained to be sensitive to the special needs of kids. And we have good senses of humor," he says.

"Our training teaches us about how children grow and develop. Learning about development is one of the most important parts of pediatrics," Dr. Palumbo adds. "We're interested in the whole child—his feelings and his interests and how he's doing in school—not just how his body is working."

Another important part of being a pediatrician, Dr. Palumbo says, is prevention. These special doctors want to do more than just take care of children when they're sick. They want to teach them good health habits so that they will be able to resist sickness and avoid accidents. Pediatricians talk to their patients about having good habits such as wearing safety belts, getting enough sleep, avoiding junk food, taking part in sports, and making regular visits to the doctor.

Next time you go to your pediatrician, be prepared for the visit. Think about what you'd like to talk over with your doctor. Are you worried about anything? Are you curious about how your body works? Ask your pediatrician—he or she is an expert on how you grow and change.

Why do I have to get shots, anyway?

Your body is an amazing machine. It can protect itself from many sicknesses. Often, when it does get sick, it cures itself.

But invisible enemies called *germs* attack your body all the time. The germs live in the air you breathe, in the food you eat, and even on the surface of your skin. But don't worry—your body comes equipped with a good system to keep the germs from doing you harm.

To understand how your body's defense system works, imagine a video game. On the screen, you see a shape. It's your body. Suddenly, germs invade—perhaps through the mouth or through a cut on the knee. You've got to get rid of the germs!

To do that, you use a chemical called an *antibody.* The *white cells* in your blood manufacture these chemicals. The antibodies race around the imaginary video screen after the germs. They catch them and wipe them out. You've won! The prize is good health.

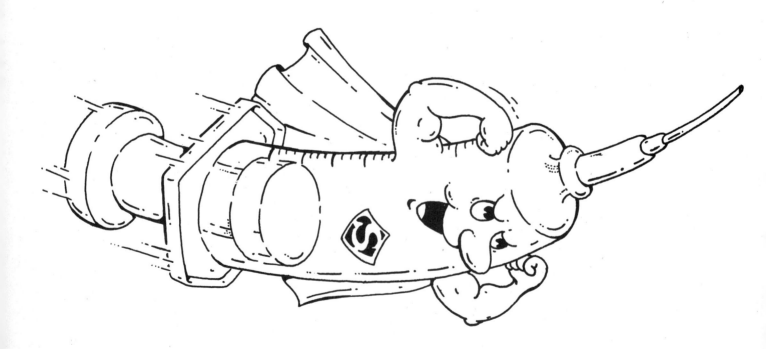

Antibodies are the weapons your body uses to fight infection and sickness. They stay in your body, ready to fight invaders at any time. The defense system is so complicated that each germ you may get has a special antibody to fight it. Once your white cells have made an antibody, it stays in your system. If the same germ shows up again—*boom!* The antibody takes care of it.

When you're born, you have some antibodies already. But you don't have enough to protect you from all the germs out there. That's where shots—also called *immunizations* or *inoculations*—come in.

Let's let a doctor explain. Dr. George Cohen works at Children's Hospital National Medical Center in Washington, D.C. He knows a lot about germs. Dr. Cohen sees many patients every day. Some of them come to him to get shots before starting a new school year.

"Germs cause certain diseases that can make kids very sick," he says. "A shot is a medicine that will help your body make chemicals called antibodies to fight these germs. It hurts for a few minutes, but then it helps you keep certain sicknesses away for a long time."

When you get a shot, the doctor puts a liquid called a *vaccine* into your body. Vaccines contain germs that have been specially treated. The germs in the shot aren't strong enough to make you sick. But they are strong enough to make your white blood cells produce antibodies to fight the germs.

Vaccines can protect you from serious illnesses such as polio, measles, mumps, and whooping cough.

When you go to your pediatrician to get a booster shot, you probably feel a bit scared. That's okay—almost everybody feels that way.

When you're getting ready to go to your doctor's office it might help to remind yourself that you're already an old pro at getting shots. By the time you were two years old, you had already received a whole bunch of shots.

You probably don't remember getting them. After all, you were just a baby. But your parents are sure to have some stories to tell you about early visits to the family doctor. They may also have a list of the shots you've already had. Ask your mother or father to show you the record of your immunizations. It will make you feel good to know that your body has been prepared for its important job of keeping you well.

My friend broke his arm on the playground. It stuck out funny, and you could tell it really hurt. The nurse took him to the emergency room. Now his arm's in a cast. What happened to him at the hospital? And how does a broken arm heal?

At the hospital, a doctor examined your friend's arm and discovered that it was painful and swollen and didn't look like his other arm. An X ray was taken to find out what was going on under the skin. The X ray helps doctors decide how to treat the break. If it's a very simple break, the next step is to apply a cast to the arm.

The doctor puts on the cast to protect the broken arm from getting hurt again. The cast keeps the bone from moving as it heals. Because the broken bone can't move, the patient feels less pain.

You can see what happens when a bone breaks by doing a demonstration with a wooden pencil. Snap the pencil in two. When you try to put the two ends back together again, you'll notice that it's very hard to make them fit perfectly. But if someone helps you, you can hold the two ends together while a partner puts putty or clay around the broken part. When the human body goes to work to repair a broken bone, it makes a substance called *healing*

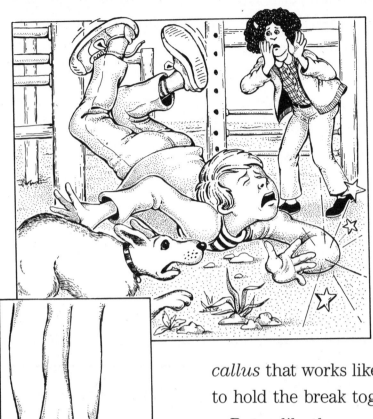

GREEN STICK FRACTURE

callus that works like the putty or clay to hold the break together.

But unlike the pencil, the broken bone doesn't end up with a lumpy bump holding it together. In time, the healing callus becomes hard and smooth, and takes the shape the bone had before it was broken. Once the healing is complete, the broken place hardly shows—even on an X ray.

Your bones, even though they're hard, are very much alive. Inside, they're light and spongy. In fact, your bones are about three-fourths water.

Doctors often see a kind of break in young people's bones that they call a *green stick fracture*. If you try to break a green, living stick in half, you'll see how the fracture gets its name. When

89

you try to snap a green twig in two, it bends. One side splits, but the other holds together. That's what happens in a green stick fracture of a bone, too. Children are more likely to get green stick fractures than adults are because their bones are still flexible and growing and contain a lot of water—like a young tree. Luckily, green stick fractures heal fast.

When a bone breaks, it starts to heal itself right away. The healing callus forms in a few hours. After a couple of days, a layer of stiff tissue has formed around the break. It makes a natural cast to hold the bone in place—in the same way that a plaster cast keeps an arm still. At the broken edges, bone cells grow toward each other and join.

This amazing repair job takes only about four to six weeks in children. Adult bones heal much more slowly. A break that puts your friend in a cast for four weeks might put an adult in one for four months.

As the broken bone heals, the doctor makes more X rays of it, right through the cast. When the healing looks complete, the doctor will hold the arm and press the place where the break was. If there's no more pain, it's time to remove the cast.

Doctors use a special tool to remove casts. It looks like a saw, and it's very noisy. It cuts through the plaster. When the doctor put the cast on in the first place, he or she covered the skin with some padding. When the cast is being removed, the doctor stops the saw when it reaches that padding. The patient doesn't have to worry that the saw will get as far as the skin.

If you're careful—and lucky—you may never experience a broken bone. But if you do, there are some tricks you can use to make wearing a cast as comfortable as possible. Turn to page 130 to find out how.

I get a lot of bruises and skinned knees. But the bruises go away fast. How does my body fix itself that way?

Minor falls can cause painful cuts, scrapes, and bruises. Luckily, the injuries aren't serious. They hurt for a while, but they heal quickly.

Here's what happens when you get a bruise on your knee, say, from bumping into something. If it turns into a black-and-blue mark, you know you've bumped hard enough to break the tiny blood vessels under your skin.

When this happens, the blood inside these vessels leaks out into surrounding tissues. The broken vessels quickly heal themselves, but the blood that leaked out stays in your tissues for some time.

At first, the banged-up place on your knee looks red. But it soon begins to turn into a black-and-blue mark. That happens as parts

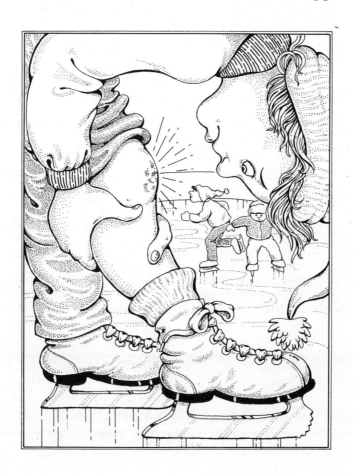

of your blood called *platelets* clump together, forming a sticky web. This begins a process called *clotting*. As your blood clots, it turns a darker color.

What you see when you look at the black-and-blue mark on your knee is the clotted blood under your skin, showing through the way a picture shows through tracing paper. If you have light skin, the bruise is easy to see. If your skin is dark, the bruise may not be as visible.

But it's still there—and it still hurts. That's because swelling around the clotted blood puts pressure on your nerves, causing pain.

Over the next few days, your nasty-looking bruise starts to fade. This happens because parts of your blood go to work to clean up the spill.

Your blood is a mixture of different parts. You've already learned about the platelets. It also contains red cells, which carry oxygen, and white cells, which fight germs. There is also *plasma*, the liquid part of the blood. Plasma contains many useful chemicals.

White cells act as a cleanup crew on the spilled blood that forms your bruise. They gobble it up. As the white cells absorb the spilled blood, the black-and-blue mark slowly disappears.

Now let's look at the other knee. Let's say you fall down and hit it on a sharp rock. You've got a cut.

When you get a cut you feel pain because tiny nerves in your skin send a message to your brain. The message says, "Something's wrong here. Send help!" Many nerves are located just under your skin, which can make a bump, a bruise, or a cut pretty painful.

But those nerve endings help you, too. They warn you to pull your finger away from the sharp point of a knife. They make you snatch your finger away from a hot stove. And they let you know when you've been cut and need to do some first aid.

If the cut you've gotten looks deep and is bleeding a lot, show it to an adult. You may need to see a doctor to have the injury stitched shut. If the cut is a small one, and if it doesn't hurt very much, you can use simple first aid to treat it.

Wash your cut off with warm water and soap. Then cover it with a clean gauze pad, and push down gently. The pressure helps stop the bleeding. Then put on a bandage to cover the cut. The bandage keeps germs from invading the cut and causing an infection. Once your cut is nicely covered, you can forget all about it and let your body heal itself.

Your body started to heal the cut, in fact, as soon as you got it. The blood flowing out of the cut carried away most of the germs that got in. White blood cells arrived to fight any germs that weren't washed away.

In the meantime, the blood in the cut started to clot. Platelets clumped together to close off broken blood vessels. Fibers in the clot shrunk together, pulling the sides of the cut closed. A scab formed.

Under your scab, new skin cells begin to grow. Your blood carries in chemicals to help build the new skin. Once the replacement skin is complete, your scab falls off. You're as good as new.

In the spring, I sneeze so much that people tease me about it. Why does spring give me allergies?

Spring brings a lot of nice things. The days get longer. Softball practice starts. It's warmer, and flowers bloom. But for a person with allergies, spring means something else, too: sneezing.

Allergy season opens as the trees begin to give off pollen. Pollen is that dusty stuff that floats in the air at this time of year. Bees love it, and trees depend on it to reproduce. But if you get hay fever, you don't need or like pollen at all.

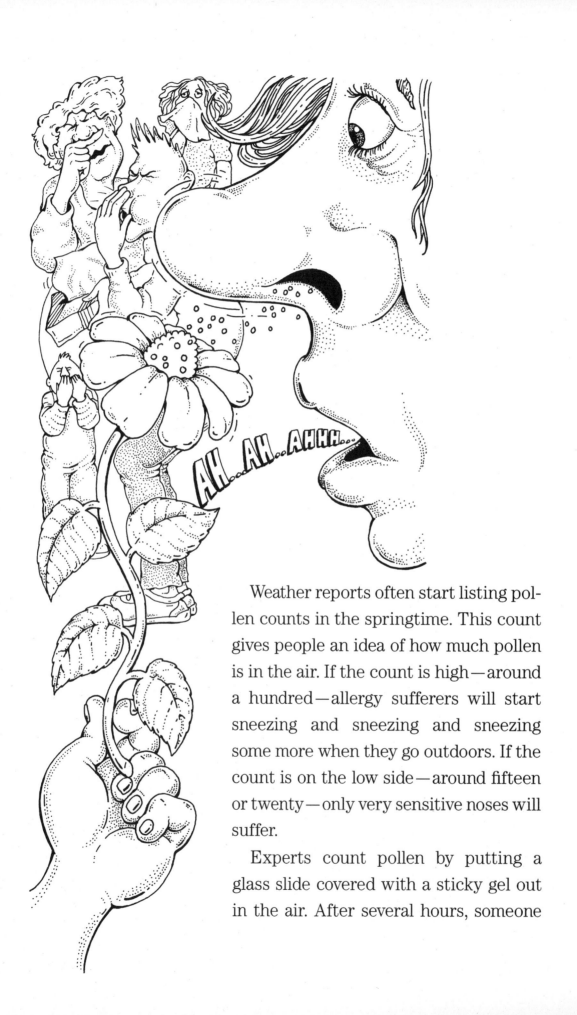

AH...AH...AHHH...

Weather reports often start listing pollen counts in the springtime. This count gives people an idea of how much pollen is in the air. If the count is high—around a hundred—allergy sufferers will start sneezing and sneezing and sneezing some more when they go outdoors. If the count is on the low side—around fifteen or twenty—only very sensitive noses will suffer.

Experts count pollen by putting a glass slide covered with a sticky gel out in the air. After several hours, someone looks at the slide through a microscope and estimates the number of pollen grains on it. That rough number is the pollen count.

In early spring, the pollens found on the slide come mainly from trees. Later in the year grasses produce lots of pollen. At the end of summer, a plant called ragweed starts causing trouble for allergic people.

When pollen gets in your breathing passages, the grains irritate the delicate tissues in there. Many people develop allergies to the bothersome grains. Allergies happen when the *immune system*—the body's defense system against germs and other invading substances—becomes oversensitive to dust, pollens, or other irritants.

Your immune system makes antibodies to fight off materials that enter your body from outside. These antibodies attach themselves to cells called *mast cells* in the lining of your nose and throat.

If you're allergic to tree pollen, your body releases antibodies when you breathe some of the pollen in. The antibodies trigger your mast cells to make chemicals called *histamines*. The effect is kind of like setting off tiny bombs inside your nose. The bombs send out chemicals that produce the swelling, itching, running nose, and sneezing we call hay fever.

Hay fever isn't a fever, and it's not usually caused by hay. But it can make you feel miserable. Its medical name is *allergic rhinitis*. Those words mean that the sufferer has a swollen nose, but the name sounds like it has something to do with a rhinoceros. When you have hay fever, your nose may get so swollen and itchy that you feel like a rhinoceros. But at least you won't be the only person feeling that way. Some 15 million people in the United States suffer from hay fever each year.

One of the most common symptoms of hay fever is sneezing. When you're riding the bus or sitting in study hall in the spring, you may notice that there's a lot of sneezing going on. Everybody seems to have a slightly different sneezing style. Some sound like explosions. Others are quieter. Some people sneeze just once. Others may sneeze more than ten times during each "fit."

When you have a cold, mucus drains and tickles your sneeze reflex. When you have an allergy, the histamines your body produces have the same effect. Because a sneeze is a reflex, you do it without thinking. You can't control it, either. You may have tried to stifle sneezes, and you probably found out that it felt as if you were going to explode.

Here's what happens when you sneeze: The muscles that help you breathe draw in a big gulp of air. Then the muscles contract, or squeeze, and force the air back out. It's an explosive and powerful movement. It pushes lots of air and drops of moisture out of your nose. And they travel fast. How fast? Scientists have clocked sneezes at 103 miles an hour as they leave the nose and mouth.

Anything irritating can cause a sneeze: cigarette smoke, a change in air temperature, even bright light. The purpose of the loud *ahhh-chooo* is to carry irritating things away. But when the problem is pollen, you just take in more bothersome grains with your next breath, and the sneeze cycle starts again.

During hay fever season, it's a good idea to carry some Kleenex with you everywhere you go. You never know when your sneeze reflex will get its next tickle.

At camp I got mosquito bites and poison ivy. They itched like crazy! Why do things like poison ivy and mosquito bites itch so much?

Your skin protects your body pretty well most of the time. But there are some things it isn't equipped to handle without swelling

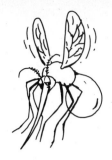

up and itching. One of these is the bite of the female mosquito.

Almost everybody is allergic to mosquito bites. When the insect bites you—and only females do—it drinks a tiny drop of your blood. In exchange, it leaves behind a tiny bit of its saliva.

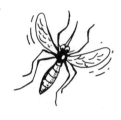

Certain things out in the world—mosquito saliva, poison ivy, poison oak, and other things—contain chemicals that cause allergic reactions in humans. You've already read about how pollen can trigger allergies.

Pollen causes allergies when you breathe it in through your nose. Mosquito saliva and poison ivy get into the body through the skin. Then the body sends the chemicals called antibodies to fight them. The antibodies cause special cells to release histamines. Then the histamines make fluid

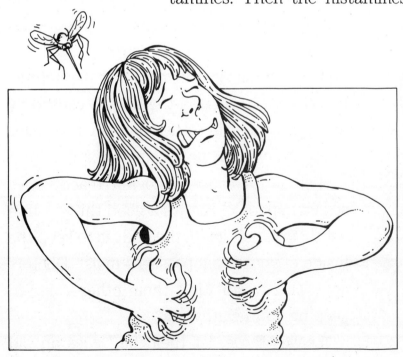

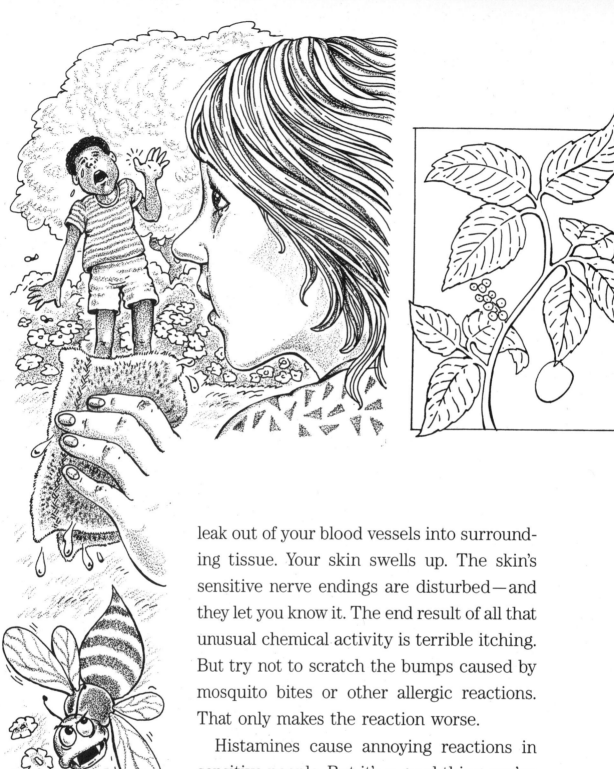

leak out of your blood vessels into surrounding tissue. Your skin swells up. The skin's sensitive nerve endings are disturbed—and they let you know it. The end result of all that unusual chemical activity is terrible itching. But try not to scratch the bumps caused by mosquito bites or other allergic reactions. That only makes the reaction worse.

Histamines cause annoying reactions in sensitive people. But it's a good thing you've got them. Their job in the body is to keep the inside of your nasal passages moist. Doctors are still investigating their other roles in keeping you healthy.

"Leaves three, let them be," goes an old

saying about poison ivy. That's good advice. But it can be hard to avoid the three-leaved plant. You may see it along bike paths, hanging from trees in the park, or even growing in your own backyard. It's a good idea to learn to recognize and avoid poison ivy.

If you do get into it by mistake, rush to the sink and wash the area where the plant touched you. Use lots of soap and water. You may be able to head off the allergic reaction. It's more likely, however, that you'll see a rash appear. It may show up in a few hours, or it may take a few days.

Poison ivy and its relatives, poison oak and poison sumac, contain an oil that sticks to anything that brushes up against them. Your bike tires, your dog's coat, or your shoes can pick up the oil. Then you may get poison ivy even if you didn't touch a plant directly.

It's a rare person who doesn't ever get the little itchy bumps these plants cause. Nearly three-fourths of the American population is allergic to them.

Once the reaction starts, you'll start wondering how long you're going to have to suffer. That's different for different people. Some are much more sensitive than others. Some cases of poison ivy clear up in a few days. Others last longer.

Some people are so sensitive to poison ivy that they have very bad reactions to it. They swell up, and they may get feverish and sick. When that happens, it's a good idea to go to the doctor for medicine to fight the reaction.

But a minor case of poison ivy can be treated with things you probably have in your kitchen cupboard. To soothe the itch, apply a paste of baking soda and water, or soak in a tub of cool water with a couple of cups of cornstarch added to it.

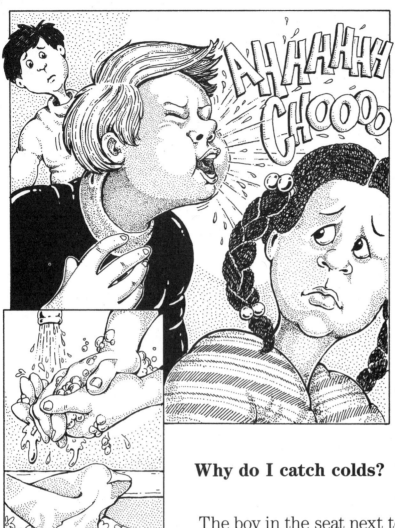

Why do I catch colds?

The boy in the seat next to you at school has a cold. *Achoo!* He sneezes—and he doesn't remember to cover his nose with a handkerchief. He rubs his nose with his hands, and later passes you a pencil you dropped.

When your classmate sneezed, he probably sent his cold germs flying all through the room. When he touched your hands, he may have passed some of his germs along to you.

There's a chance you might catch a cold, too. Most kids catch from two to six colds a year. In fact, colds are one of the sicknesses children get most often.

Scientists have found cures for many of the illnesses people catch, but they still haven't discovered a cure for the common cold.

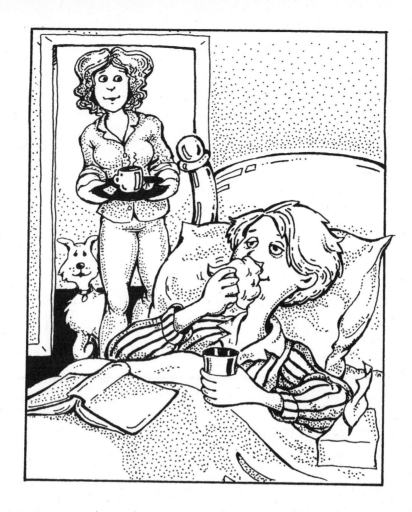

Colds are caused by viruses—tiny invisible germs. More than two hundred different cold viruses have been found. That's a lot of different ways to get the sniffles and sneezes. If you catch one kind of cold and get over it, you can still catch another kind. That's why you may catch several colds each year.

Luckily, colds aren't usually very serious. But you may feel, look, and sound miserable for about a week before you get better.

Colds cause the upper respiratory tract—the part of you that does your breathing—to swell. The wet lining of the tract, called the mucous membrane, becomes wetter than usual. Your nose starts to run.

The insides of your nose, mouth, throat, and ear passages are all connected. You may notice this more than usual when you have a cold. You get a runny nose. Fluids run down your throat, and along with the virus make it scratchy and sore. You may start coughing. Your ears may feel funny, too.

Kids catch the largest number of colds between September and May. That's when you spend the most time cooped up indoors. It's easier to be exposed to germs in closed-up, heated spaces.

Getting too tired, being very, very busy, or eating a poor diet may make you more likely to get sick. But even if you sleep well, stay happy, exercise regularly, and eat a balanced diet, you probably will still catch at least one cold during the school year.

What can you do when that happens? Not much.

Americans spend half a billion dollars each year on cold medicines. These medicines may help the *symptoms* of a cold, such as sneezing and coughing. But they don't cure the sickness.

When your grandmother was a little girl, her mother probably made her rest and drink lots of juice and soup when she caught a cold. Today, those old home remedies are still a good idea.

When you blow your nose during your cold, you lose fluid from your body. It needs to be replaced. Just as a driver makes sure there is enough water in a car's radiator to keep it running smoothly, you need to drink enough water to keep your body's engine running well, especially when you have a cold.

So if you do catch a cold, remember to drink liquids and get plenty of rest—and you can look forward to getting well soon.

Why does the flu make people feel so awful?

Flu, or *influenza,* is caused by invisible germs called viruses. When an influenza virus gets into your body it begins to multiply. The harmful germs attack your cells, making you feel sick. You may get a headache, body aches, and chills and fever when you have the flu. You may feel as if all you can do is sleep. You may have

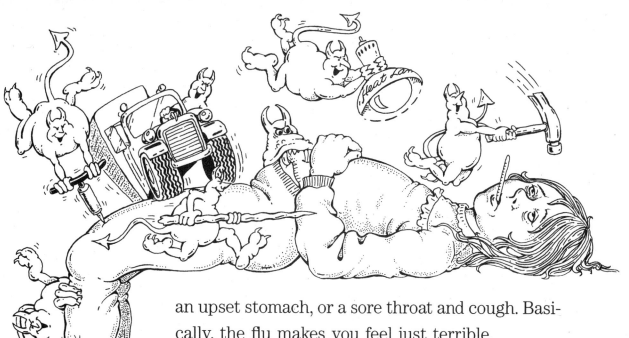

an upset stomach, or a sore throat and cough. Basically, the flu makes you feel just terrible.

Some of those awful feelings are signs that your body is hard at work trying to get rid of the attacking flu virus. Doctors think that when a slight fever raises the temperature inside your body, it creates an environment viruses don't like. Higher temperatures might make it harder for some viruses to multiply once they get into the body.

But viruses also directly cause fevers. As they multiply, they produce chemicals called *pyrogens*. Pyrogens interfere with the part of your brain that controls your temperature. Normally, your body stays at about 98.6 degrees Fahrenheit. It's the job of a part of the brain called the hypothalamus to check on the temperature of your blood and keep it at a safe level.

The substances released by viruses can temporarily confuse the hypothalamus. Instead of setting the temperature of the blood at normal, it sets it higher—at 100 degrees, or even 102 degrees. When your fever gets that high you feel strange, but

103

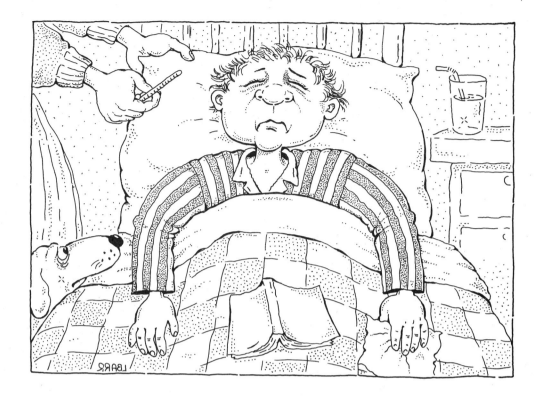

you're not really in danger. But when a fever gets extremely high—over 105 degrees—it's time for the doctor to do something fast. Fevers that high can damage your cells.

If you had the flu, your temperature might hover around 100 or 101 degrees for a few days. You'd feel weak—too weak to even watch TV, probably. You'd be glad to stay in bed. You'd sleep a lot, and drink a lot of liquids. You wouldn't take aspirin, though. Aspirin and flu are a dangerous combination that can cause a really serious illness called Reye's syndrome. Instead, your doctor would tell your parents to give you an aspirin substitute to ease aches and pains.

Staying in bed is important when you get the flu. While flu itself is not usually considered a serious illness, it can have complications. Old people or people who are weak because they have heart conditions or lung problems sometimes develop pneumonia after they catch the flu. Pneumonia is a serious condition that causes swelling of the lungs. Pneumonia can be dangerous, especially for people who are already weak from another illness.

Because of the possible danger of complications, people in high-risk groups usually get flu shots in the winter so they can avoid getting sick from the virus. Developing the medicine that goes in flu shots can be hard for doctors to do, though. As flu viruses multiply, they also change slightly. By the time the medicine for a shot has been developed to ward off one form of flu, another form of the virus may have shown up. The flu shot protects people from the old form of the virus, but not from the new form.

Many doctors insist that grown-up people in high-risk groups get flu shots. Your grandparents or people you know who have chronic illnesses that make it hard to fight off disease probably get the shots.

If you don't get flu shots, don't worry. Many pediatricians feel that flu shots aren't necessary for their healthy patients. Your doctor will decide whether or not you should receive the shot.

How can I get rid of headaches?

If you watch much television, you've probably seen dozens of advertisements about headaches. The ads show grown-ups describing their headaches, telling how much they hurt, and where the pain is located. They moan and groan and complain. To judge from TV, you'd think grown-ups have headaches all the time.

Lots of people do get headaches. They can be caused by tension, by stress, by emotional upsets, or by illnesses such as colds and the flu. Some people get headaches from eating certain foods such as cheddar cheese or peanuts. Headaches are no fun. But luckily they're usually not very serious.

Kids often get headaches, too. A study of nine thousand chil-

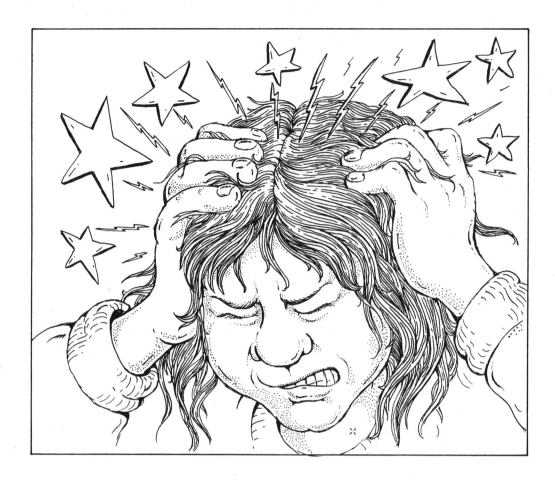

dren in Scandinavia showed that about half of them reported getting headaches every now and then. About one in ten of the children got bad enough headaches to check with the doctor about them. The study also showed that kids tend to get more headaches more often as they grow older. Four-year-olds had fewer headaches than fifteen-year-olds, for example.

Kids may get headaches from staying out in the sun too long, watching TV for hours on end, losing sleep at a slumber party, or from having a fight with a friend or family member. Being anxious about getting a lot of homework done or worrying about a test can bring on a headache, too.

Headaches may be a sign that a cold or the flu is on its way. Getting a mild bump on the head—say while playing on a jungle gym or after a fall from a bicycle—can also cause a brief headache.

Even a sudden change of temperature can bring on a headache—as you may have discovered if you've gotten an ache in your head after wolfing down an ice cream cone too fast. As you can see, headaches are a common problem.

Some doctors feel that learning relaxation techniques can help relieve headaches. Next time you feel a headache getting started, you might give this method a try. It's easy. Just breathe deeply and close your eyes. Imagine a pleasant situation that makes you feel happy and relaxed—such as lying on a blanket under a tree after a picnic in the sun on a warm summer day. This simple relaxation exercise might help you feel better.

Headaches are often caused by tension in the head and neck muscles—the ones you use to smile, frown, shake your head, chew, and so on. Sometimes these muscles get too much use. For example, when you have a big fight with your best friend, your emotions may cause the muscles in your head and face to contract, or squeeze tight. This stimulates your nerves, and the next thing you know you've got a headache. Lying down for twenty minutes might help ease the pain. Making up with your friend might cure the headache, too.

Almost all the headaches that kids get are easy to cure. But every now and then, a child may get a headache that doesn't go away after resting and taking aspirin or an aspirin substitute. Sometimes a headache sticks around for more than an hour after someone gets a hard bump on the head. If a headache is so bad that the child who has it wants to lie down, or feels like throwing up, it's a good idea to tell an adult about it and maybe call the doctor.

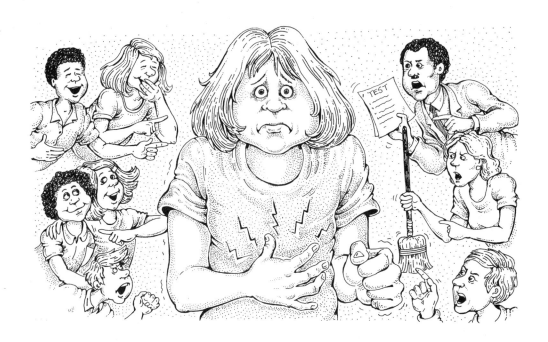

**My mom and dad say they have something called "stress."
Do kids get stress too?**

Kids do experience stress. This story will explain what stress is.
You may have had the same kinds of things happen to you.

Ann had to take a math test, but she was absent from school the
day it was given. She said she had a stomachache, but when she
went to the doctor, nothing was wrong.

Ann's teacher called to check on how she was feeling. "I think
she's okay," Ann's mother said. "But she seems kind of worried
lately. I think she's under stress."

Stress is your body's response to the tensions of daily life. Some
stress is always there—it keeps you alert and aware, ready to face
the challenges of the day such as remembering to take your books
and keys to school in the morning, studying for a test, or trying to
win that softball game. But when life gets very busy, when major
changes happen, or when things aren't going too well in a family,
there can be too much stress.

Some grown-ups would laugh at the idea that kids can experience stress. They think that being a child is all fun and no worries or work. But Dr. Marvin Fine, a psychologist at the University of Kansas, says stress in kids is no joke. In addition to teaching at the university, Dr. Fine advises elementary and high school teachers about how to handle student stress.

Dr. Fine says that some kids feel like failures and get depressed if they can't do perfect work in school. When kids are worried or depressed, they use up energy they could be using for learning and having fun.

School is only one of several things that can cause stress in kids, Dr. Fine says. Moving to a new school or town, leaving old friends, moving to a new house, or having a new brother or sister can cause stress, too.

Stress is a part of everyday life. From the moment the alarm clock goes off in the morning until you go to bed at night, you run into different kinds of pressure. There's pressure to get to the bus stop on time, to get the right answers on the spelling test, to be included in the kick ball game on the playground, to clean up your room, to finish your homework before your favorite TV show starts. If things don't go smoothly, you can get nervous, upset—even sick.

You can't completely get rid of stress in your life—and you wouldn't want to. "A little stress can help some people perform tasks more efficiently," says Dr. Fine. Think about when you get "psyched up" for a test, for example. You may feel nervous, but that feeling of excitement can help you do your best job.

But for people who have a hard time with stress, that feeling of excitement can interfere with doing things well. These kids may avoid situations that are stressful. In class, kids may be "there physically, but not mentally," Dr. Fine says. Daydreaming through math class can be a way of avoiding stress.

When stress becomes a problem, kids sometimes become anxious and unhappy. They may withdraw from their friends and family, start having trouble sleeping, and behave badly in school. They may have trouble eating, or get upset stomachs easily.

Ann's stress upset her stomach. She was feeling so worried about math that it was literally making her sick. The odd thing was that Ann was very good at math—so good that she couldn't accept the fact that she made mistakes sometimes. She got really mad at herself if she got even one problem wrong.

The math teacher felt bad that her student was so upset about the test. She and Ann sat down and had a conference. "Everyone makes mistakes," the teacher said. "Making mistakes can be an important part of learning. I was a terrible speller in school—but I survived."

Dr. Fine suggests that students who experience stress try relaxation techniques to get through the bad experience. The next time Ann had a math test, she started to get a panicky feeling when she saw the paper. Her stomach started to hurt, too. But she closed her eyes, reminded herself that she didn't have to get a perfect score, took a few deep breaths, and started again.

Ann did a good job on the test. She missed one word problem, but her parents and her teacher were pleased with the test anyway. "Maybe I'll get through fourth grade after all," Ann thought.

5

GROWING UP

From the time before you're born until you're very old, your body keeps changing. This chapter answers some questions about how those changes happen, and why you grow up to be the particular human being you are.

Why do I have a belly button?

It's time for your swimming lesson, and you arrive at the pool in your bathing suit. As you wait on the edge of the pool for the signal to dive in, you suddenly notice that some of the kids in your class have belly buttons that stick out a little. But your navel goes in, like a small dimple in the middle of your stomach. Another swimmer has one that's practically flat.

What's up? Is something wrong with your navel—or is it the other guy who has the problem?

You're all okay. Each kind of navel you see as you wait to go swimming is normal. They formed during the first few weeks after birth. But they actually got started a long time before that.

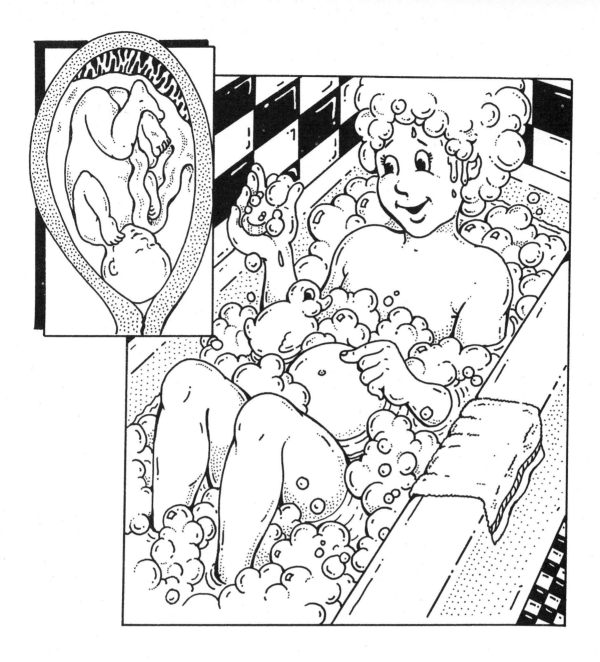

You spent about nine months living inside your mother's body before you were born. Have you ever wondered how you got the food you needed to grow while you were living in her *uterus*, or womb? After all, you couldn't go out for a hamburger. And have you ever wondered why you could survive inside without air to breathe?

When you were a *fetus*, or unborn baby, you received nourishment from your mother's blood. Her body shared the food she ate with you. That's why your mother was probably very careful about what she ate during her pregnancy. She knew the nutrients she consumed were also helping you grow strong and healthy.

To reach your growing body, nutrients and oxygen passed from your mother through a twisted tube called the *umbilical cord*. This cord contains two large blood vessels. At one end, the tube was connected to the middle of your body. At the other end, it was attached to your mother's body.

During your mother's pregnancy, the nutrients you needed passed from your mother's body through the blood vessels in the umbilical cord, and reached you. Your cells soaked up everything they needed to grow.

As cells use nutrients, they produce waste products. These products must be removed from the body. Some of the blood vessels in the umbilical cord carry waste products away from the developing baby.

It might help to understand this process if you think of the umbilical cord as a two-way street. You can imagine that one lane is jammed with food trucks delivering nourishment to the growing baby. In the other lane, garbage trucks busily drive away, carrying waste products away from the baby.

The umbilical cord you depended on for food and oxygen developed very early in your mother's pregnancy. As you grew, the cord was at work all the time. But once you were born, you didn't need the cord anymore. Your lungs started working, and you began eating on your own. So what happened to that lifeline you used to need?

In the delivery room right after you were born, a doctor or nurse put a clamp on the cord quite close to your stomach. Then the cord was cut. This didn't hurt because the cord doesn't have any nerve receptors in it. When you came home from the hospital, you still had a small piece of the cord sticking out of your stomach. If you have a baby brother or sister, you may have seen one of these.

Before long, the leftover cord dries up and falls off. It leaves a scar behind—a kind of reminder that you were once attached to your mother. That scar is your belly button—though your doctor might call it by its fancy medical name, the *umbilicus.*

Different people develop different kinds of belly buttons after their umbilical cords fall off. That's because of the different ways the cords were attached before birth.

Some fetuses have cords that meet the skin of their abdomens in a neat line. Those babies grow up to be people with flat belly buttons.

Some umbilical cords don't quite meet the skin on the fetus's stomach. A short piece of skin called a membrane attaches the cord to the baby. These babies end up with belly buttons that collapse into their stomachs a little—the kind of belly button you probably call an "inny."

Other fetuses have a little bit of extra skin on their stomach, which grows up around the end of the umbilical cord. These babies grow up to have belly buttons that stick out a little—or "outies."

We have a new baby, but all she does is sleep, eat, and cry. When will she start acting like a kid?

If you have a new baby in your house, you already know a lot about how they behave. You know that babies may not seem to be very active in the first few months of their lives. But they're actually busy learning and growing from the very beginning.

Newborn babies are completely dependent on other people for survival. At birth, humans can't sit up, talk, walk, or feed themselves. The only way they can let others know what they want is by crying. During the first month of life a baby's neck muscles aren't strong enough to support its head. That's why you have to support the head very carefully when picking up or holding a newborn.

But babies very quickly learn to do things on their own. During the second month of life, babies begin to develop *motor skills.* This is the ability to control movement: turning the head from side to side or reaching out a hand to grab something.

Babies begin to notice other people and to interact with them very early. Next time you meet a three-month-old baby, try smiling at it. Once the baby is used to you, he or she may smile back. Getting a baby to smile at you gives you a great feeling.

By the time the baby is about five or six months old, it can turn over in bed. Parents get very excited the first time a baby turns over in its crib by itself. Ask your mother or father about the first time you did it.

By the time babies are toddlers, at around eighteen months, they can walk and run, laugh and play, get angry, feed themselves, and even say a few words and phrases. They have done an amazing amount of learning and growing in a very short time.

So much goes on during infancy that many scientists spend their whole careers studying just that part of the human life cycle. Some researchers study how babies learn language. Others focus on what a baby's facial expressions show about what it's feeling. Others concentrate on how babies learn to walk. Some researchers are interested in the kinds of relationships babies have with the people around them.

One thing researchers have proved beyond a shadow of a doubt is that babies need to be touched. Of course they also need to be fed, clothed, and kept warm and clean. But they need to be cuddled and loved. Cuddling a baby makes an older person feel good—but for the infant it's even more important. Some scientific research suggests that babies who experience a lot of physical affection grow up to be happier, healthier people than babies who don't get much hugging.

Why are some people twins? And why do some twins look alike, while others don't?

"Even our parents mix us up sometimes," says Susan, a third-grader. Susan and her sister, Pam, are identical twins. They look so much alike that they can fool their friends and teachers about which one is which. If you know them well, you can tell them apart because Pam has pierced ears and Susan doesn't. Or is it the other way around?

"We don't look alike," says Tommy, who's in fifth grade, "but our teachers are always calling us by the wrong name anyway. They sometimes just call us 'twin,' which makes me feel really mad." Tommy and his brother, Bobby, are fraternal twins. You can tell they come from the same family, but they don't look exactly alike.

What's the difference between these two sets of twins? It all started before they were born.

A human baby grows from a tiny egg cell, or ovum, inside the mother's body. To start the journey toward becoming a person, the egg must join with a sperm cell from the father. When the two cells join, they produce a new kind of cell called a *zygote*.

Both the ovum and the sperm cell contain many instructions for

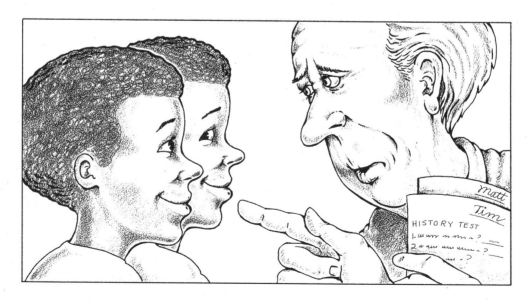

telling the baby how to grow. These instructions are contained in chemicals in the cells. Together, the cells carry enough of these instructions to produce all the characteristics of a new human being.

This recipe for a new person is contained in tiny threads called *chromosomes*. An ovum has twenty-three chromosomes. A sperm cell has twenty-three, too. Together, they make forty-six— exactly the right number to start building a person.

The chromosomes carry bits of chemical instructions called *genes*. Genes control many things about what a human being will look like. Will the baby have red hair or brown? Will it have an upturned nose? What shape will its earlobes be? The genes decide these things.

Since a baby gets half its genes from its mother and the other half from its father, it usually ends up looking like a combination of its parents. But there are so many possible combinations of genes that each human being looks unique.

Wait a minute—what about identical twins? They look alike because of an event that takes place soon after the ovum and sperm join. The zygote splits into two parts, each containing a complete genetic recipe for a new person. This is a pretty unusual event. Only about one zygote in two hundred fifty splits in two and develops into identical twins. Because the genetic instructions for each developing baby are the same, the babies will look identical, and be the same sex.

Fraternal twins, on the other hand, develop from two separate egg cells that joined with two separate sperm cells. The babies develop together inside their mother's body, and share the same birthday. They may both be girls, both boys, or a boy and a girl. Like ordinary brothers and sisters, they'll share certain family characteristics. But they weren't produced from identical genetic recipes, so they won't look like mirror images of each other.

Fraternal twins aren't quite as rare as identical twins—they happen in about one pregnancy in one hundred fifty.

Sometimes a mother gives birth to three babies, called triplets. Sometimes there are even more babies, but multiple births like these are very rare.

After twins are born—whether they are identical or fraternal—they grow into two individual people. Some identical twins may have a hard time convincing other people that this is true. Are there any pairs of twins in your school? Make an effort to treat them as separate and unique people rather than as "the twins." They'll appreciate it—and you'll make two special friends.

Twins' parents can help them feel like special people, too. "Sometimes my parents take me out by myself," says Pam. "We talk about things that interest me. Then the next week they do the same thing with Susan. It's neat."

"It's a lot of fun to be a twin," says Bobby. "But I do get tired of people thinking that because Tom likes swimming, I must like it too. I like reading! We're both individuals."

How did I get to be a boy instead of a girl?

When the egg from your mother's body and sperm from your father's met inside your mother's *reproductive tract*, the sperm fertilized the egg—an event called *conception*—and a baby—you!—started to grow.

The blueprint for a new person has forty-six chromosomes in the zygote, arranged in pairs. Scientists who study these "genetic blueprints" call some chromosomes "X" and some "Y." The twenty-third pair of chromosomes determines what sex a baby will be.

The father's sperm is in charge of determining whether you're a boy or a girl. That doesn't mean your dad decided with his mind. It was a matter of chance, not choice. When you were conceived,

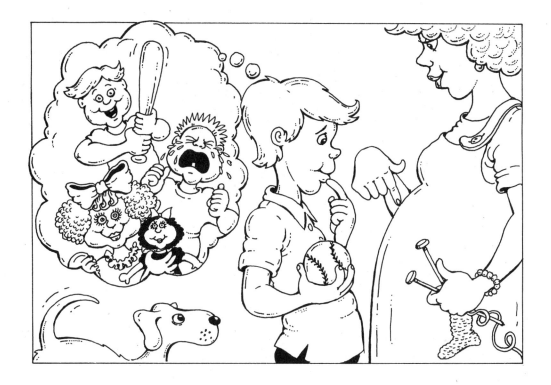

your father deposited millions of sperm cells within your mother's body. Only one sperm cell was needed to fertilize her egg. The mother's ovum always contributes an X chromosome to the twenty-third pair. If the sperm cell contributes another X chromosome to the twenty-third pair, making an XX, the baby will be a girl. If the sperm cell contributes a Y to the twenty-third pair, the baby will be a boy. If you're a boy, the twenty-third pair on your genetic blueprint was an XY pair.

Why are a lot of the boys shorter than the girls in my class at school?

It's normal for girls to be taller than boys at a certain time in their lives. That's because females start their *growth spurt* earlier than males do. For girls, this period of fast growth occurs somewhere between age nine and sixteen. Around age twelve is the most common time. For boys, the growth spurt occurs between age

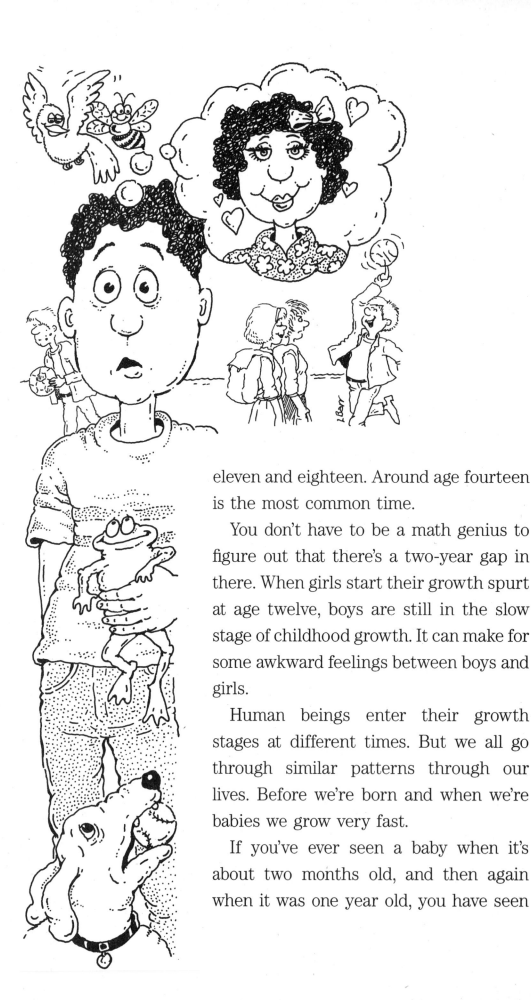

eleven and eighteen. Around age fourteen is the most common time.

You don't have to be a math genius to figure out that there's a two-year gap in there. When girls start their growth spurt at age twelve, boys are still in the slow stage of childhood growth. It can make for some awkward feelings between boys and girls.

Human beings enter their growth stages at different times. But we all go through similar patterns through our lives. Before we're born and when we're babies we grow very fast.

If you've ever seen a baby when it's about two months old, and then again when it was one year old, you have seen fast growth in action. During the first year of life, infants grow one and a half times as tall as they were at birth, adding about 10 inches to their height. They sprout another 10 inches between the ages of one and four. Then growth slows down. During the elementary school years, kids grow more slowly—not much more than two inches a year.

Each person grows at his or her own pace. It's important to remember that when you read the growth charts in your doctor's office. You may grow faster or slower than the "average" person. But that doesn't mean there's anything wrong with you.

Whenever your growth spurt starts, you need to take good care of yourself. The rapid changes in your body can make you tired and irritable. You may find it hard to concentrate in school. You may find that little things upset you more than they used to. And your clothes don't fit anymore.

You need additional rest and lots of good food during this period of your life. Your body has work to do; if you're a boy, you'll grow somewhere between 8 and 12 inches in a two-year period after your growth spurt begins. If you're a girl, you'll grow almost as much.

During the growth spurt, glands in the body produce substances called hormones. Hormones are chemical messengers that tell cells that it's time to grow and change. One gland, the *pituitary*, produces the hormones that control how fast you grow, and when the spurt stops.

Doctors at the Krogman Growth Center in Philadelphia say that following a few commonsense rules can help you grow to your full height. First, make sure you get enough sleep. Lack of sleep can slow the growth spurt down. Get regular exercise, and eat lots of protein foods such as fish, eggs, cheese, and meat. And don't worry! Even if your growth spurt starts late, you'll soon catch up to your friends.

I'm almost a teenager. Why are my feelings and my body changing all of a sudden?

Julie, Bob, and Diana are all in the same sixth-grade homeroom. The three of them grew up in the same neighborhood, so they've known each other for a long time. When they were little, they used to ride tricycles together. They all played for the same co-ed softball team during the summer. They walked to school together, and helped each other with their homework. They were good friends.

But lately, Julie, Bob, and Diana have had a problem. As they approach their thirteenth birthdays, their feelings about all kinds of things have gotten confused. Sometimes, Bob likes Julie a lot—in a way he didn't like her before. He gets nervous around her, and acts dumb and shows off. Julie just ignores him. But Diana has started to like Bob in a new and different way, too. She thinks about him a lot, but when she sees him she feels shy and gets really quiet, even though she has known him all her life. Diana feels really mad because Bob likes Julie better than he likes her.

What's going on here?

The situation these young people are in happens to many, many kids as they get older and reach *puberty*. You may have had confusing feelings like Julie's, Diana's, or Bob's yourself. Going through puberty isn't easy.

During puberty, human beings pass from childhood into young adulthood. Many physical changes accompany puberty. The body grows taller and changes shape. Both sexes begin to develop body hair. Boys' shoulders broaden, and they develop more muscles. Girls' hips grow broader, and their bodies become more rounded. Girls develop breasts, and begin to menstruate. Boys' sex organs get larger. These changes help prepare the body to have children

122

someday. Boys develop faint mustaches—a signal that they'll be shaving soon.

The physical changes of puberty happen gradually, and at different times for different people. Some kids enter puberty around age ten or even earlier. Others don't begin to notice changes until they are into their teenage years. It's normal to start puberty early or late. When it happens depends on the individual's own biology.

At puberty, the pituitary gland, located in the brain, sends hormones into the bloodstream that trigger the ovaries in the female and testes in the male to make the hormones that cause the physical changes described above. These hormones also cause the body to perspire more and bring about changes in your skin. You may notice that you sweat more under your arms, and you may develop pimples. Hormones also make your voice change. Both boys' and girls' voices change during puberty, but it's more noticeable with boys.

Emotional changes come with puberty, too. The confusing feelings about the opposite sex that Diana, Bob, and Julie experienced are common during puberty. It's also common to feel embarrassed or uncomfortable about the changes your body goes through.

There's not much you can do about puberty—it just happens. The uncomfortable part of it is no fun. But the physical and emotional changes of puberty are a sure sign of something exciting—growing up. During puberty you will become more independent. You'll start thinking for yourself more and making more of your own decisions.

During puberty, it can be hard to communicate with adults. You may feel as if they don't understand you, or that they don't take your feelings seriously. Sometimes it's hard to ask your parents or other adults about the changes you're going through. At this time of your life, you may find your friends are more sympathetic than older people are. After all, your friends are going through puberty, too.

Why do I get bumps on my face?

Getting older has its advantages. But it can cause problems, too. A common complaint teenagers make is about their skin. Puberty causes pimples. Yuck!

Pimples happen when your *sebaceous glands,* which are designed to keep your skin soft and supple, begin to produce too much oil. The extra oil plugs up pores—tiny holes in the surface of your skin. You can see your pores if you look closely at the skin around your nose or on your forehead.

When the pores get clogged with oil, bacteria move in. They

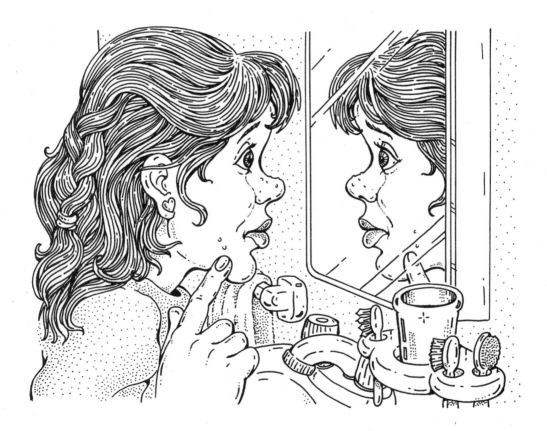

thrive in the area, but they make the skin look red and swollen. Pus develops, forming a pimple.

Why do you get pimples when you're an adolescent, just when you want to look good? It doesn't seem fair. But the hormones that cause the physical changes of puberty also cause the sebaceous glands to work overtime. As your hormone production levels off, the pimples will disappear, too. In the meantime, wash your face with mild soap two or three times a day, and rinse with cold water to close your pores. When your pimples bother you, try to remember that you're not alone. In the United States, about three-fourths of kids between age twelve and seventeen have skin problems of some kind.

What happens to people as they get old?

Have you had a birthday lately? As each year passes, you probably feel more and more amazed at how *old* you're getting.

With each passing year, your body has changed. You have grown from a tiny baby into a healthy child. Soon you'll be a teenager, and then an adult. You'll get taller, heavier, and stronger. Eventually, you'll stop growing, and start aging.

How did your body know how to grow bigger and stronger? Your glands produced hormones that told your cells to soak up lots of nutrients. With that nourishment, your bones became longer and harder. Your muscles grew, and you got stronger and better coordinated. Your body changed shape, and will continue to change until you reach adulthood.

By the time you're about twenty-one, you'll be completely grown up. All of the systems you'll need to be a healthy adult will be in good working order. If you eat well and get lots of rest and exercise, you'll probably feel terrific and go on feeling that way for many, many years.

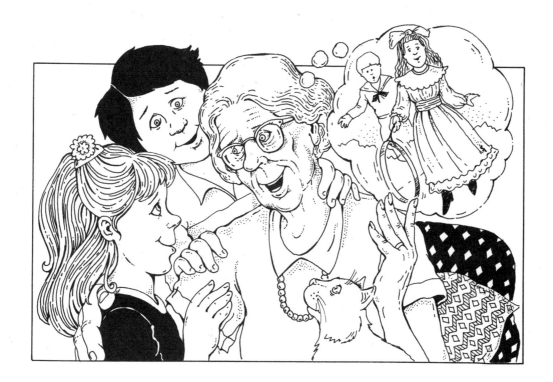

Eventually, you'll begin to grow old. You probably know some elderly people. They may be friends, neighbors, or members of your family. When you spend time with them, you may notice that they move more slowly than younger people do. They may not hear or see as well as they used to. They may be more likely to catch illnesses than younger people are. All of these changes are part of growing older.

If you know any older people well, you also know that although they may not be able to move as fast as you can, or see as far, that they have a lot to offer you. If you have a great-grandmother, she's probably over eighty. She can probably tell you stories about her childhood that will amaze you.

The difference between the bodies of young people and old people has to do with their cells. A human body contains trillions of cells of many different kinds. As you learned at the very beginning of this book, cells are the basic building blocks that make up your blood, your muscles, and your brain—in fact, every part of you.

As you move and grow, your cells experience a lot of wear and tear. But that's okay, because they can repair themselves. As you get older, though, your cells are less active, and less able to protect themselves from the stresses of daily life.

When older people's skin cells wear down, their faces grow wrinkled. As cells in their hair stop producing pigment, or color, their hair turns gray or white.

Today, doctors have developed lots of ways to help aging people feel better and healthier in spite of their years. In the United States, people can expect to live healthy, productive lives for at least seventy years. Many Americans live—and feel well and happy—much longer than that.

Activities

HOSPITAL CARE PACKAGES

When your friends are in the hospital, it's important to keep in touch with them. Getting better is more than a matter of taking medicine and getting a lot of rest. A sick person needs support from friends and family, too.

It can help a hospitalized child a lot if classmates and friends send pictures they've drawn or postcards, or maybe even projects that the patients can do in bed. Things to decode, secret messages, and crossword puzzles are a lot of fun. If your friend is in for a long stay, send games in more than once.

Telephone calls can help, too. It may not be a good idea to call in the evening. Some children's hospitals don't allow calls after eight in the evening, but a call in midafternoon can be great. Remember that hospitalized kids may not want to talk long, depending on how they're feeling. But even a quick hello is a reminder that you're thinking about your friend.

You may be wondering why you can't visit your friend. School-

128

age kids are exposed to all kinds of germs every day. Just think of how many kids in your class have had a cold or the flu this year. It's usually a good idea to limit a hospitalized child's exposure to germs. After all, he or she is in the hospital to get better, not to catch a cold.

SUNBURN TIPS

Before going outside, apply sunscreen to all the parts of your skin that will be in the sun. That means the soles of your feet, the tips of your ears, and the part in your hair. (A sunburned scalp can really hurt!) Always put sunscreen on again after you go swimming. And don't be fooled by a cloudy day. The harmful rays of the sun can get through cloud cover and burn you just as badly as they would on a sunny day.

TASTE TEST

This experiment will show why a stuffed-up nose makes eating less enjoyable.

The way a food smells is an important part of the experience you have when you eat it. You can find this out by doing a simple experiment with a partner. Cut and peel small pieces of several fruits and vegetables. You could try apple, potato, pear, peach, cucumber, carrot, turnip, or celery. Ask your parents which fruits and vegetables in the refrigerator are okay to use for your taste test. Ask for permission to use the knife, too.

Now close your eyes and hold your nose tightly. Have your partner place each piece of food on your tongue in turn, and bite down on it. Without opening your eyes or letting go of your nose, say what the food is. Have your partner write your answers down.

Next, repeat the experiment with your eyes still closed, but without holding your nose. Don't bite down on the food this time—see if you can identify it just with your taste buds. Again, name the food and have your partner write down your answer.

When you compare the two lists, you'll probably see that you got more right answers when you used taste and smell to guess the food. Your taste buds are pretty sensitive—but your nose helps you taste, too.

ON THE PULSE

When you're sitting down and relaxed, put two fingers over your wrist. When you have found your pulse, say "go" and start counting. Have someone else time you for 30 seconds. Multiply the number you get by 2. That's your resting pulse. In young children, the resting pulse will be between 90 and 120 beats per minute. In older kids and adults, the resting pulse will be somewhere between 60 and 80 beats per minute.

If you take your pulse when you're exercising, you will get a higher number of beats per minute. The heart may beat as many as 200 times per minute during really hard exercise. That's because your muscles need more oxygen when they're working hard, so the heart speeds up and you breathe deeper to keep up the supply.

It might be fun to try taking your pulse in lots of situations. Then you'll know the times your heart works its hardest. Try taking a pulse when you first get up in the morning, after you take a bath, in the middle of a spelling exam, when you feel tense, after you ride a bike, after you see a scary movie. You can think of other situations on your own.

CAST COMFORT

These tips come from Dr. Richard Reff, a bone specialist at Children's Hospital National Medical Center in Washington, D.C.

- Don't let your cast get wet. If the padding between the skin and the plaster gets wet, Dr. Reff says, "it's like wearing a wet sock for about three weeks."
- Don't put anything inside the cast to scratch the skin. Being in the dark for a long time makes the skin very sensitive, and if you scratch it, it won't heal well under the cast. Also, if the padding inside the cast gets wadded up, it can cause painful pressure—sort of like walking with a stone in your shoe.
- Blow warm air into the cast using a hair dryer on the lowest setting. This will soothe itchy skin.
- Use a large plastic bag to cover the cast if you go outside on a rainy day, or when you take a bath or a shower.

GOING THUMBLESS

This experiment will make you appreciate your thumbs in a way you never have before. Do it with your family, some friends, or a class. Compare notes when you're done.

Have someone wrap adhesive tape around both your hands so that your thumbs are securely taped to the sides. Your fingers should be left free. Then try to go about your daily tasks. You'll be surprised.

Here's what one group of kids discovered when they tried this experiment one summer day: You can't play badminton, because it's hard to grip a racket when you don't have a thumb. It's also hard to throw the birdie in the air accurately. It's almost impossible to keep a secure hold on an ice cream cone. It's no fun to go to the pool for a swim when you can't unbutton your shirt when you go to the locker room to change into your suit.

What will *you* discover when you go "thumbless"?

BUILD A STETHOSCOPE

Your doctor uses a device called a stethoscope to listen to your heartbeat. Maybe you have had a chance to hear it, too. If not, ask your doctor to let you listen next time you go for a physical.

You can listen to someone's heart by using a much simpler device than a stethoscope. Take a cardboard tube left over after you use up the paper towels or plastic wrap in your kitchen. Ask a friend to stand still, and then place one end of the tube against the upper left side of his or her chest. Put your ear to the other end of the tube. You should be able to hear your friend's heartbeat. That regular *lub*-dub, *lub*-dub means that the heart muscle is busy keeping the body supplied with oxygen.

Or, you can make a pretty good stethoscope with some rubber tubing and a funnel. Both items can be found in hardware stores, or you may have them around the house. Just slip the end of the rubber tube around the neck of the funnel. Apply the large end of the funnel to your "patient's" chest. Listen through the rubber tube attached to the small end. You'll hear the heart thumping away.

Every minute of every hour of every day of your life, your heart pumps blood. The sound you hear—*lub*-dub, *lub*-dub—is the muscle working.

AVOID ACCIDENTS

Thousands and thousands of children are hurt in accidents every year. Accidents are the number-one killer of children aged one to fourteen. Many of these tragedies could have been avoided, doctors say.

Now you know why your parents are always telling you to be careful. They try to protect you as much as they can, but they're not always right beside you to watch out for things that might cause you harm. Sometimes you have to take care of yourself—and your younger brothers and sisters or friends. These guidelines should help.

- Be safe and careful when you are on the playground. Remember not to twist swings, swing empty seats, or walk in front of a moving swing. Be extra careful when climbing. You could hurt yourself or somebody else.
- When you ride your bicycle, obey all traffic signals. Wear a protective helmet, and don't ride after dark. Also, don't ride an older person's bike. A bike that's too big for you can be dangerous. So can trying to give your friends a ride on your bike.
- If you are going to be outside playing as it gets dark, make sure you wear light-colored clothes that will reflect automobile headlights. That way, you'll be seen by an oncoming car.
- If you are at home with your brother or sister and your parents aren't home yet, always call for help if you get scared or if someone gets hurt. For example, if you are playing and someone falls and hits his head, don't be afraid to call for help even if you're not sure it's an emergency. Know a neighbor's phone number and the number of the police and rescue squad.
- Know how to escape in case of a fire in your house. If you see a fire or smell smoke, get out of the house fast. Don't stop to get a jacket or try to put out the fire. Close doors as you leave, and crawl out of the house if there is smoke in the air: fresh air is near the floor. Call the fire department from a neighbor's house.
- Whenever you ride anywhere in a car—even just a few blocks—wear your seat belt.

Afterword

This book has answered many questions about how your body works, and why you feel the way you do. But if you are a curious kind of person—and most kids are—there may be other things you want to know about your body. There's a person you see fairly often who can probably answer some of the questions this book didn't get to. He or she can also tell you about things this book does explain, but in more detail.

Who is that person? Your doctor. He or she is a great source of information about health and nutrition, fitness and feelings. Talking things over will help you learn, and will help your doctor get to know you better. You'll find out more about your body, and your doctor will discover that you're an interested patient who wants to take an active part in staying healthy for a lifetime.